The Wheatgrass Book

Other Avery books by Ann Wigmore

BE YOUR OWN DOCTOR
THE HEALING POWER WITHIN
THE HIPPOCRATES DIET AND HEALTH PROGRAM
RECIPES FOR LONGER LIFE
THE SPROUTING BOOK
WHY SUFFER?

The Wheatgrass Book

Ann Wigmore

AVERY PUBLISHING GROUP INC.

Wayne, New Jersey

The medical and health procedures in this book are based on the training, personal experiences, and research of the author. Because each person and situation is unique, the editor and publisher urge the reader to check with a qualified health professional before using any procedure where there is any question as to its appropriateness.

The publisher does not advocate the use of any particular diet and exercise program, but believes the information presented in this book should be available to the public.

Because there is always some risk involved, the author and publisher are not responsible for any adverse effects or consequences resulting from the use of any of the suggestions, preparations, or procedures in this book. Please do not use the book if you are unwilling to assume the risk. Feel free to consult a physician or other qualified health professional. It is a sign of widsom, not cowardice, to seek a second or third opinion.

Cover photo by Martin Hochberg
Cover design by Martin Hochberg and Rudy Shur
Text illustrations by Linda Deming
In-house editor Diana Puglisi
Typeset by House of Equations

Library of Congress Cataloging in Publication Data

Wigmore, Ann, 1909-
 The wheatgrass book.

 Bibliography: p.
 Includes index.
 1. Wheatgrass (Wheat)—Therapeutic use. 2. Vegetable juices—Therapeutic use. 3. Food, Raw—Therapeutic use.
 4. Health. I. Title.
 RM255.W54 1985   613.2'6   84-24194
 ISBN 0-89529-234-3 (pbk.)

Printed in the United States of America
10 9 8 7 6 5 4

Contents

This book is dedicated to the improvement of human health and the prevention of illness, through an understanding and appreciation of wheatgrass juice and its value as both food and medicine.

Foreword

Wheatgrass juice is fast becoming the most popular "new" health and diet food in America. In actuality, however, this sweet green juice pressed from young wheat plants is not new—it was first applied to human health by Ann Wigmore, founder of the Hippocrates Health Institute, over thirty years ago. Since then, more than half a million glasses of wheatgrass juice have been consumed at the Hippocrates Institute in Boston alone!

Ann Wigmore has used wheatgrass juice on a daily basis for three decades. At the age of seventy-five, she is the epitome of health and vitality. She is constantly on the go, lecturing, traveling, and writing—often about wheatgrass juice. For as she points out in this book, fresh wheatgrass juice is an ideal food for anyone who wishes to prevent illness and improve his or her health.

While wheatgrass juice is rapidly increasing in popularity, many people lack an awareness of its proper role in a healthful lifestyle. *The Wheatgrass Book* is the most complete and authoritative guide to the subject of using wheatgrass juice for maximum benefit. The fresh juice of young wheat plants is a storehouse of natural vitamins, minerals, chlorophyll, enzymes, and life energy. In this book, you will learn how wheatgrass juice helps to nourish every cell of the body, and cleanse them of toxins. It is perhaps the safest and most effective way to healthfully supplement your diet.

During the last sixteen years I have had the privilege of administrating several popular wholistic health centers in the

United States and Europe. As executive director of the Hippocrates Institute, I have witnessed many complete reversals of
symptoms. I attribute these to the remarkable regenerative
power of wheatgrass juice and live foods (the uncooked
sprouts, greens, vegetables, fruits, nuts, and seeds that are
part of the Hippocrates Diet and Health Program).

A few years ago, with the encouragement of India's former
prime minister, Morarji Desai, and the assistance of prom-
inent physicians such as Dr. G. Datey, M.D., Ann traveled to
India to establish a number of healing camps, where she ad-
ministered wheatgrass and live foods to hundreds of sick and
malnourished men, women, and children. She has published
dozens of articles reporting the amazing rate of recovery ex-
perienced by many of these people.

In the United States, the effectiveness of wheatgrass and
live foods in preventing illness has been praised by Dr. Arthur
Robinson, the director of the Oregon Institute of Science and
Medicine. In 1978 at the Linus Pauling Institute, Dr. Robinson
completed a research project in which wheatgrass and live
foods were fed to mice with squamos cell carcinoma. In Dr.
Robinson's words, "The results were spectacular. Living foods
[including wheatgrass] alone decreased the incidence and
severity of cancer lesions by about 75 percent. This result was
better than that of any other nutritional program that was
tried." Dr. Robinson is presently conducting a research project involving Hippocrates Health Institute guests.

Over the years, many guests at the Hippocrates Institute
have requested that Ann write a concise book about wheatgrass juice. I am happy to say that *The Wheatgrass Book* has
been worth waiting for. It is filled with practical information
about growing and using wheatgrass. In addition, this book
summarizes the most interesting medical research on wheatgrass juice. I'm sure you'll enjoy reading *The Wheatgrass
Book* as much as I have, and I'm sure that your first refreshing drink of wheatgrass juice will be your start toward a more
satisfying and healthful lifestyle.

Brian Clement
November, 1984
Boston, Massachusetts

Preface

The Wheatgrass Way to Super Health and Beauty

We walk over it, lie down on it, mow it once a week during the summer, and knock little white balls into holes cut in it, but the thought of *eating* grass seems absurd. Unless you happen to be the winner of the Kentucky Derby, or Aunt Nellie's prize heifer, you probably have never entertained the thought of chewing on a bunch of grass. And if you haven't visited the Hippocrates Health Institute, chances are that you have not tried wheatgrass juice.

In this book I hope to persuade you to consider using wheatgrass and its juice as food, medicine, and an overall tonic for various ailments. Whether you suffer from chronic fatigue, sinusitis, ulcers, or a more serious illness like cancer, wheatgrass chlorophyll extracted from seven-day-old wheat sprouts may help you even where other medicines have failed. Of course, nothing can replace a sound diet, exercise, and a positive attitude in keeping you in top shape. But wheatgrass can give you energy and strength to help you gain better control of your health.

Chlorophyll, the green juice of grasses, has been valued since biblical times. Grass has been used as a folk medicine remedy by many people around the world. During the First World War, I began to learn about its remarkable healing properties. My grandmother used grasses to heal wounded soldiers in the European village where I was born. I came to America to live with my parents while I was still a child. It wasn't until about thirty years later, during the early 1950s, that the memories of my grandmother's use of grasses and other plants resurfaced as a result of personal health problems.

I began my own experimentation with wheatgrass and other grasses on animals. Wheatgrass proved to be the fastest and easiest variety of grass to grow. The wheatberries used to grow it were (and still are) inexpensive and easily obtained. Moreover, wheatgrass turned out to be favored by my pets. It worked miracles for their well-being (I will show you how you can use it to help your pets live longer and in better health in Chapter 8), yet I still doubted its usefulness for human health. So I expanded my study of grasses, focusing on wheatgrass in particular.

I contacted my friend and associate Dr. G. H. Earp Thomas for his expert opinion of the potential usefulness of wheatgrass for human health. A soil and plant scientist, Dr. Thomas had prior knowledge of grasses and chlorophyll. Yet after a few weeks of chemical analysis and library research, he was quite surprised to find that wheatgrass contained many vital nutrients which he felt could serve as regenerative and protective factors in human health. According to his findings, fresh wheatgrass juice was theoretically capable of sustaining human health and life for weeks or even months at a time. Dr. Thomas also came across some research papers written by Dr. Charles Schnabel, who advocated the use of young wheat and other grasses in animal and human nutrition. Schnabel estimated that fifteen pounds of wheatgrass was equal in protein and overall nutritional value to three hundred and fifty pounds of ordinary garden vegetables. I will speak more about the nutritional content of wheatgrass in Chapter 5.

The real proving ground was my own body, which was sickly and weak after twenty years of living and eating as an average American. A few weeks after I started chewing and juicing young blades of fresh wheatgrass, and eating fresh sprouts and greens, a festering case of colitis that I had suffered with for months began to improve. The problem, which is particularly difficult to remedy with conventional medical treatments, eventually cleared up entirely.

My energy level soared and I felt well again. I *knew* that wheatgrass was a powerful invigorator of the body. To prove to myself that it would also help others get well I began delivering fresh wheatgrass juice to a number of bedridden ill and elderly people in my neighborhood. I was amazed at the results. In a matter of weeks, all of them were able to get out of bed, and they became more active than they had been in years.

I'm sure that much of the degeneration and illness we suffer from today is brought on by the lack of vitality and life in the food we eat. Most food that Americans eat is overcooked and half-dead (for example, 100 percent of the enzymes in food are destroyed by cooking). Beverages are loaded with sugar, alcohol or stimulants that create an illusion of energy which fades quickly as the day wears on. In contrast, the nutrients in wheatgrass and raw foods such as sprouts, fresh vegetables, fruits, nuts, seeds, and Hippocrates Diet preparations made from them, are not destroyed by cooking or processing. These *living* foods can restore vigor and energy to an ailing, tired body.

For years, at the Hippocrates Health Institute in Boston, we have been witnessing a transformation in our guests—they arrive worn out and run down, and return home vitalized and full of pep.

An analysis of blood samples drawn from more than two hundred Hippocrates guests before and after the two-week program gave scientific support to our observations. Performed at the Arthur Testing laboratory by Thelma Arthur, M.D., the study showed that within two weeks of following the Hippocrates *live food* Diet and drinking wheatgrass juice, the blood is detoxified and the immune system is strengthened. Both of these changes lead to more energy and an improved ability to combat and reverse illness.

Wheatgrass is not only healthful, it's easy to grow and easy to use. With a handful of wheatberries, some water, a tray filled with an inch of topsoil, and a cover, you can grow your own wheatgrass in just seven days—at a cost of about ten cents a tray. If you can't grow the grass yourself, you can probably buy it locally from someone who does, because there are wheatgrass and sprout growers in almost every major city in the U.S. and abroad.

A tray of wheatgrass yields about seven to twelve ounces of juice (depending upon the size of the tray). Once you get some juice (about one to four ounces at a time will do) all you have to do to get its health benefits is drink it. Some people enjoy the taste, but even if you dislike it at first, you will love the way you feel within a few minutes—and for hours later.

In addition to drinking wheatgrass juice, there are dozens of other ways you can benefit from it. For example, wheatgrass juice can be used as a scalp treatment for lusterless hair, or as a cleanser, astringent, and tightener for all types of skin. Several drops in each nostril will help to clear blocked sinuses, and a few ounces in your bath water or rubbed into your skin will stimulate healthy circulation and give you a warm glow. But that's not all. True to my childhood memories of wounded soldiers becoming well through the use of grasses, wheatgrass helps heal cuts and bruises faster, and draws poisons out from deep inside the body so they can be eliminated.

Who can benefit from using wheatgrass? Anyone. Whether you're overweight or underweight, have a tendency towards anemia or are afraid of cancer, wheatgrass can help. In this book I will show you how you can use wheatgrass for cleansing and healing your body, improving your diet and appearance, and preventing illness.

In addition I will share my discovery of the wheatgrass fast, a shortcut to better health and weight loss that combines wheatgrass and chlorophyll-rich "green drinks" with special cleansing techniques. Finally, you will also find some delicious recipes that are popular favorites at the Institute. Have you heard of a Grasshopper? Wait until you try your first Wheatgrasshopper (see page 89)!

One question I'm often asked is, "Do I have to change my diet totally in order to benefit from wheatgrass?" Of course not. However, I do feel that for the best possible results you should follow the Hippocrates Diet of raw, living foods as closely as you can. I also recommend that you use fresh wheatgrass rather than dehydrated or tablet forms. These serve as a good source of dietary fiber, but they carry with

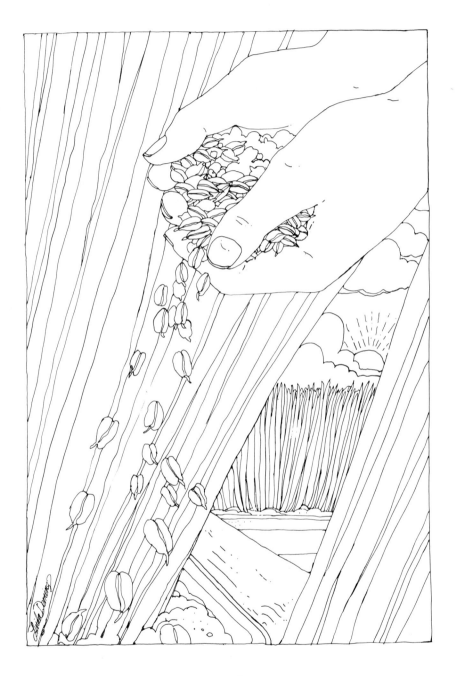

Thriving Wheatgrass

them little of the life force (enzyme power) found in fresh wheatgrass juice. In fact, at the Institute we suggest that you juice wheatgrass immediately after you cut it, and drink or use it right after you juice it, thereby getting the maximum benefit of its enzyme life forces.

From the juice bars of California to the health spas of New York, wheatgrass is fast becoming one of the most widely used supplemental health foods. After years of experience of working with wheatgrass, it is my feeling that if you begin to use fresh wheatgrass juice on a regular basis, you will gain a bounce in your step, a better physique, an improved complexion, and a sparkle in your eyes. And it is my hope that your use of wheatgrass juice will help to move the medical establishment toward more research on this valuable nutritional and health aid.

1

Green Power From Wheatgrass

The greatest service to any country is to add a useful plant to its culture.

Thomas Jefferson

Wheatgrass can help you get more from your life—more energy to be active, more confidence in your ability to stay healthy, and more hours alert and awake each day to accomplish your goals in life. I am assuming you are reading this book because you feel there is room for improvement in your health. Maybe you get worn out easily, wake up tired or in pain, or can't manage to drop those ten extra pounds by the end of the spring anymore. In any case, you're probably right: there is room for improvement in your health and wheatgrass juice could be your route to a healthier, happier life.

MORE ENERGY

Millions of Americans, young and old, are drained of their energy by the end of a day, despite the fact that most of them walk less than two blocks and sleep eight to ten hours. Many middle-aged people accept the loss of youthful energy as an inevitable product of aging. I used to feel that way, but that was before I discovered wheatgrass and raw foods.

Do we have to settle for less energy at any age? I haven't, and you don't have to either. Long-lasting fatigue is abnormal and is largely caused by a poor diet. Modern life demands a great deal of energy which cannot be adequately replenished by a nutritionally imbalanced diet. While a certain amount of fatigue after a long day of work is normal, when a night's rest doesn't leave you perfectly refreshed and recharged, there is a problem. If you wake up looking and feeling as tired as when you went to bed you are not getting what your body needs from your diet—or you are getting too many things you *don't* need and they are blocking your flow of energy. Wheatgrass can help you restore a high energy level in two ways. First, by fulfilling nutritional deficiencies, and second, by removing wastes that clog your cells, blood, tissues, and organs.

Each of us is the keeper of over ten trillion little batteries called cells. Like flashlight batteries, our cells hold a charge of electricity. In order for this charge to be strong and steady we need to have a steady supply of the proper nutrients, especially the high-quality minerals, vitamins, enzymes, and amino acids contained in wheatgrass juice. With the addition of wheatgrass and raw foods to your diet, your cells will store a maximum electrical charge, and you will have plenty of energy. At the same time, wheatgrass will help to release excess fats, mineral deposits, and proteins that are trapped in the organs of digestion and elimination, and in the blood, thus saving you energy that would otherwise be spent in your body's struggle to cleanse itself.

WHEATGRASS CAN LENGTHEN YOUR DAY

One thing you may notice right away after beginning the wheatgrass and raw (live) foods regimen is that you will need less sleep than you do now. Six hours of sleep—maybe even less—is adequate as long as it is deep and undisturbed sleep. Even though many people sleep in excess of eight hours a night, their sleep is chaotic and broken up by raids on the refrigerator and trips to the bathroom. These people often wake up feeling and looking exhausted.

During sleep, the body goes on "automatic" and balances and re-energizes its cells. Ideally, a night's sleep of four to six

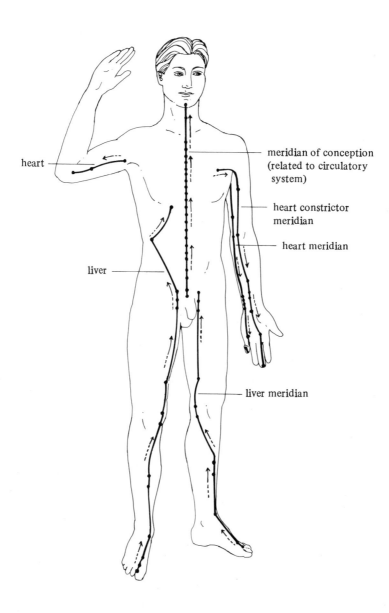

Energy Flow Through Body

hours, and an optional afternoon nap of an hour, will give your body plenty of time to renew and refresh itself. But when your body is overloaded with food, more than half of it consumed at the evening meal, your sleep will be more restless and less restful. Whenever your cells are more out-of-balance, as often occurs during an illness, the more sleep you will need.

Wheatgrass and other raw foods are light, clean foods that nourish and cleanse the body, whereas red meats, cheeses, and sugared and processed foods are heavy and tend to congest and age our cells. After a few days of drinking and applying several ounces of wheatgrass juice, if you avoid heavy, clogging foods, your body's housecleaning burden will be reduced and one morning you will awaken from a short, deep, undisturbed sleep refreshed and renewed. As accumulated wastes and debris are removed, you will find that your energy and confidence will return.

REVERSING ILLNESS

Wheatgrass juice is perhaps the most powerful and safest healing aid there is. Not because it can attack and destroy bacteria or malignant cells, like some drugs, but because it has the ability to strengthen the whole body by bolstering its immune system. The exact way in which wheatgrass juice improves the state of the immune system is not yet known. Rather than there being one or two "elements" responsible for the healing power of wheatgrass, I feel strongly that the key factor is a unique combination of nutritional values, chemical values, and energetic attributes.

The body's ability to fight illness is determined by the immune system. Through improving the health of the immune system, wheatgrass juice and other raw foods may increase the odds of your overcoming any kind of health problem. In contrast, modern drugs are taken to correct one symptom or another without effectively strengthening the overall state of health. In reality no drug has ever healed a person. Knowing this full well, Hippocrates, the father of medicine, stated, "The body heals itself; the physician is only nature's assistant."

The unique nourishing and cleansing properties of wheatgrass, combined with the grass juice factor (which I will discuss later on), make it an ideal ally in the battle against disease, including illnesses like heart disease and certain forms of cancer, especially those that lead to depressed immune response and the subsequent attack of the body by microbes or viruses. For anything, including wheatgrass and other raw foods, that strengthens the body and especially the immune system, can serve only to increase well-being.

PROTECTION FROM CITY BLUES

Nearly every day one group of scientists exposes another chemical as a dangerous carcinogen, while another group of specialists creates one. Our air is unfit to breathe, our water too acid and polluted to drink, and thousands of acres of our topsoil are eroded each year. Many cities which were once the lifeblood of culture and the arts are slowly becoming huge concrete and electronic wastelands where people spend their days before hurrying home to the suburbs at night. But even in the suburbs, industrial pollution, auto exhaust, and toxic chemicals have taken their toll. It seems that unless we experience a major environmentally-based technological revolution, pollution and its attendant health risks will be here to stay.

Fortunately, there is a sensible way to combat the "city blues." We can protect ourselves from environmental hazards by strengthening our internal defenses. If our eliminatory processes work more efficiently, toxins that do enter the lungs and blood won't stay as long. Poisons that do linger can be more easily neutralized by a healthier liver. With fewer heavy foods in the diet, we can increase the amount of oxygen in the blood and ease the burden on the circulatory system. Then pollution will affect us less severely than it will strike people who remain heedless of their health. There is even evidence (which I will discuss in more detail later) that wheatgrass can protect us from both low- and high-level radiation.

In this age of mass information and telecommunication, few things have been kept a secret for as long as wheatgrass juice. Things are changing, however. The past few years have seen the first significant research on chlorophyll and wheatgrass since the 1940s, and all of the reports I have studied confirm that wheatgrass is a top-notch cleanser, builder, healer, protector, and rejuvenator of health. Few foods or medicines contain as many active live ingredients as wheatgrass. We cannot deny the fact that without wheatgrass and the other grasses that cover the earth, the human race could never have survived. Nor can we turn our backs on the amazing potential of wheatgrass as a superfood and medicine that is completely safe in any amount, and available to everybody for just pennies a day.

2

Green For Life

Fifty million years ago our guardian angel, the grass, arrived to our planet—to make life possible, and to prepare the Earth for the human race.

Edmond Bordeaux Szekely

Maybe you take the springtime, with its myriad of green and the physical and mental relief it gives you, for granted. Or perhaps you are too busy chasing after paper to notice the green trees and grasses that grow in your back yard. But chances are, somewhere deep in your mind you remember that plant life on earth is responsible for your existence here. Without the miracle of photosynthesis, there would be little warmth, air for us to breathe, or food to eat. I have come to the conclusion that the further from our conscious minds this memory is, the closer we come to failing as a civilization.

In this chapter I will discuss the importance of green plants in our ecosystem and how chlorophyll, the "blood" of a plant, is related to human blood. The nature of chlorophyll itself, and the relationship between modern agriculture and nutritional deficiencies will also be discussed.

When we stop appreciating the green life—the trees, grasses, and plants that we call nature, we tend to abuse them—to our detriment. Where green life has been effectively extinguished, in inner-city ghettos and prisons, mental illness and violence are commonplace.

The residents of Los Angeles have known of the importance of green plants and trees for years. "Tree People," a Los

Angeles-based conservationist group, estimates that if it were not for the millions of trees and green plants, many cities would be uninhabitable due to pollution. The Tree People have been commissioned by the state of California to plant one million "smog resistant" trees, as many of the existing trees are dying due to pollution.

In Japan, researchers have concluded that the amount of oxygen required to support the people and industry in that country far exceeds the amount supplied by green plants there. If it were not for the steady supply of oxygen generated by the Amazon jungle of South America, and distributed by wind currents, countries like Japan could suffer from a shortage of oxygen. The jungles of the Amazon are being rapidly depleted for use in making paper and other wood products, thus reducing the total oxygen content of our atmosphere. We cannot afford to forget that the quality of the air we breathe and the climate we live in are determined by green plant life *everywhere*.

PLANT BLOOD

You could say that green plants are to the earth as the lungs are to humans and animals, except they work in reverse. That is, plants "inhale" carbon dioxide and "exhale" oxygen, whereas humans and animals exhale carbon dioxide and inhale oxygen—a perfect symbiotic relationship.

Years ago, Dr. Hans Fischer and a group of associates won a Nobel prize for their work on red blood cells. During their research, the scientists noticed that human blood, which carries oxygen to all our cells, is practically identical to chlorophyll on the molecular level. In the human body, red blood cells are characterized by the oxygen-carrier, hemoglobin, which has as its central nucleus the mineral element iron. Most green plants, on the other hand, are characterized by chlorophyll, which has magnesium as its nucleus. A careful examination of the two molecules shows them to be strikingly similar (see illustration).

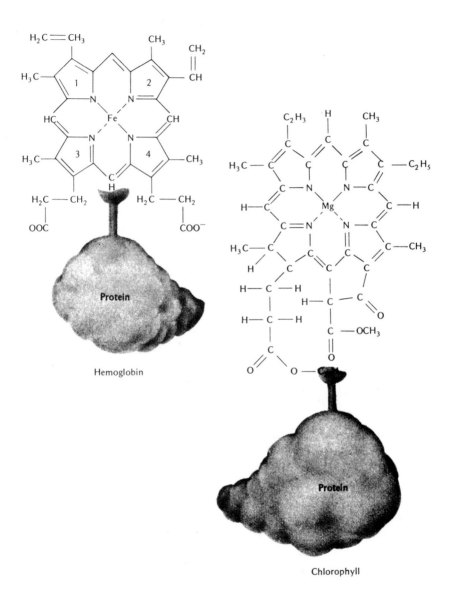

A Comparison of Chlorophyll and Hemoglobin

In 1930, Dr. A Zin showed that an injection of chlorophyll increased the red blood cell count of animals with normal hemoglobin counts. Scientists J.H. Hughs and A.L. Latner of the University of Liverpool went one step further. In their study, reported in the *Journal of Physiology* in 1936, a number of animals were made anemic by daily bleeding. After their hemoglobin levels were reduced to less than half the norm, the animals were divided into ten groups. Five of the groups were fed various types of chlorophyll in their diet. The five groups of control animals did not receive any chlorophyll. Those animals receiving "crude" or raw, unrefined chlorophyll were able to increase the speed of hemoglobin regeneration by more than 50 percent above average, to approximate their previous blood values in about two weeks. However, the group receiving synthetic chlorophyll showed no improvement in the speed of hemoglobin regeneration. In their report, the scientists concluded: "It seems, therefore, that the animal body is capable of converting chlorophyll to hemoglobin." Raw, unrefined chlorophyll seemed to be the best for this purpose.

Chlorophyll was formerly used by some physicians to treat anemia. But even if you're not anemic, an increase of red blood cells could mean better circulation and oxygenation to the cells, and rapid body cleansing. My empirical evidence has shown this to be the case. And since oxygen is quickly used up in the many body functions it is responsible for (the brain alone uses about 25 percent of the available oxygen in the body), the infusion of it into the blood via wheatgrass juice, among other things, stimulates an improvement in the immune system—our natural means of preventing and healing illness. In other words, the blood becomes richer and the body healthier by its use.

CHLOROPHYLL

You may be wondering exactly what chlorophyll is. Very simply, it is a green (sometimes purple) pigment found in growing plants. It contains mineral and proteinous compounds. As I mentioned earlier, it is the blood of the plant. But, like Dr. Bircher, founder of the famous Bircher-Benner clinic in

Switzerland, I think about chlorophyll in another way—as condensed solar energy.

The leaves of plants convert sunlight into energy that is stored in the plant fibers. People who have the habit of eating meat or drinking milk are merely getting this solar energy secondhand, after the cow has converted it into milk or flesh. Seventy percent of the solid matter in wheatgrass juice is crude chlorophyll. In wheatgrass (and in uncooked fresh vegetables, sprouts, and greens), you can get "concentrated sun power" firsthand.

Dr. Bircher was outspoken on the therapeutic value of green juices extracted from green leafy vegetables and grasses: "Chlorophyll," he said, "increases the function of the heart, affects the vascular system, the intestines, the uterus and the lungs. It . . . [chlorophyll] is therefore a tonic which, considering its stimulating properties, cannot be compared with any other."

The very same power that enables the roots of trees and clumps of grass to push their way through cement sidewalks in a matter of days is available to our bodies, now, in the form of wheatgrass and other green juices. The lack of this vital force is responsible for our ills today. No matter how we may neglect green plants in our diet and our lives, we will never erase our need for them from our instinctive memories—and our physiological systems.

THE NEW GREEN REVOLUTION

Many people are looking to the science of the future for answers to their problems, but as funding for basic research is dwindling, and more and more research becomes oriented towards industry, can we really trust science to guide us in our life from day to day? No doubt we owe a great deal to the scientific achievements of the past hundred years, but as our environment becomes increasingly polluted and the death rate due to cancer continues to climb, the only hope we have is to make our bodies stronger and healthier. No amount of library research or medicine will give you a stronger, healthier body. Only a good diet with plenty of raw green foods and wheatgrass, moderate exercise, and a positive and caring attitude will do this.

Thanks to the much-praised "green revolution," we have in recent decades seen greater yields of a larger variety of plants. While this green revolution is well-intentioned, the agricultural techniques that we call "revolutionary" and "improved" involve much short-sighted thinking, and bring limited positive results in terms of human health. Much of the increased crop yields are squandered on animals produced for slaughter, and the effect modern industrialized agriculture has on our topsoil is devastating. Moreover, chemical fertilizers, pesticides, and herbicides have detrimental effects on our bodies.

The new green revolution which I have been advocating for years is a more personal one. It is all about bringing green plants, grasses, and foods into your home and life. We eat so few green vegetables, fruits, and raw foods that it is astonishing that we continue to survive. Most of our food is processed with chemicals. In 1977, the United States had the dubious distinction of becoming the first nation in history whose people consumed more than 50 percent of their diet as processed items. This experiment with processed foods is dangerous; it has created epidemic proportions of degenerative diseases, many of which are labeled "incurable." In light of this fact, how can we be so arrogant as to believe that we can improve on nature? Clearly what we need today is a new green revolution. One that is concerned not only with replenishing nature's trees and green plants, but also with cleaning out the "national bloodstream," using fresh green foods and wheatgrass juice to do so.

MODERN TOPSOIL AND MINERALS

The soil we grow our food on should be a very real and serious concern to us. Not only is our topsoil eroding by the thousands of acres each year, but it is losing its vitality, just as we are losing ours. When the mineral content of the soil is poor, it yields crops that are deficient in nutrients. Without vital soil to grow food on, farmers have come to depend increasingly on various fertilizers and chemical sprays to keep their weakling plants alive.

The color and taste of fresh foods reflects the mineral value of the soils used to grow them. Would you ever dare compare tomatoes, corn, cucumbers, or any other vegetables shipped into your area out of season on an equal basis with locally grown foods? Even a gourmand knows the difference between a vine-ripened local garden tomato and the ones available in the markets during the winter. The natural red of beets, orange of winter squash, and green of kale or grass becomes richer and deeper when the soil is inherently balanced and vital. Unfortunately, in many cases, fruits and vegetables are artificially colored. These items usually have little taste and aroma.

Chemically treated fruits and vegetables which are deficient in flavor, aroma, and color can be likened to an obese person who has gained weight on excess fat and carbohydrates—bloated with water, yet containing less minerals and vitamins than normal, healthy-sized individuals.

Where will we get our minerals from in a healthful diet? Certainly not from processed foods, meats, sugar, white bread, or butter. Our best source of supply is from *organically grown* land vegetables and sea vegetables (especially the deep green varieties), and from sprouts and wheatgrass.

Organic growers are part of the new green revolution. They do not use synthetic fertilizers, herbicides, or pesticides, but rely instead on crop rotation, composting of crop residues, and a number of biologically safe measures to control insects, weeds, and other pests. Organic farmers encourage soil fertility by enriching its stores of natural minerals, earthworms, and soil enzymes. Foods grown on organic soil are balanced foods, which foster healthy, balanced people.

In recent years, however, many people who are not fond of vegetables have turned to supplemental minerals that can be dangerous and chaotic inside the body. A much better solution, if you dislike vegetables, is to juice them and drink the juice, and to use wheatgrass juice. Since wheatgrass and other green plants are among the best dietary sources of minerals, there will be less of a chance that you will come up short on any of the essential minerals if you do so.

THE ENDURING ACCOMPLISHMENT OF BARBARA MOORE

A few years ago I listened intently to news reports of Barbara Moore, who was about to set off from San Francisco on her way to New York. What attracted my attention to the story was the fact that she was walking—she expected to reach the Big Apple just forty-five days later—and that she would eat little more than grass and weeds all the way.

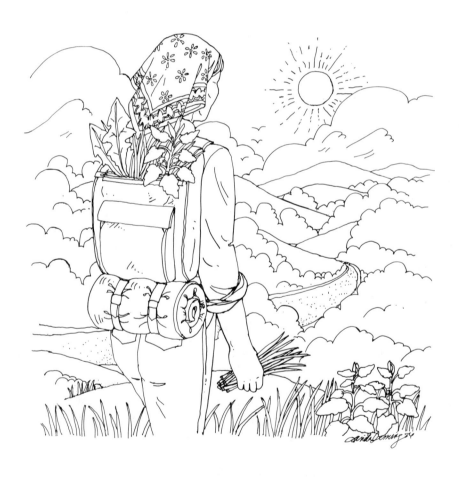

Barbara Moore on Mountain Hike

For years, Barbara Moore had made a habit of traveling to Switzerland to walk in the Alps. During many of her long treks there she subsisted on grasses, weeds, and water from melted snow. She also completed a walk across England (some one thousand miles), maintaining a five to six mile per hour pace for sixteen to eighteen hours a day. At fifty-six years of age, Mrs. Moore shattered the common belief that we need meat and lots of cooked foods to be strong and have plenty of endurance.

The day she departed from San Francisco on her grueling transcontinental "walkathon," reporters saw her carrying a banana and a jar of celery juice, the only supplements she would add to her diet of wayside grasses and edible weeds. Forty-six days later, Mrs. Moore arrived in New York, greeted by an entourage of friends and surprised reporters.

3

How Wheatgrass Chlorophyll Works

Until man duplicates a blade of grass, Nature can laugh at his so-called scientific knowledge.

Thomas A. Edison

Many theories about the active ingredients of green plants have been offered over the years. However, while we are not totally sure as yet why chlorophyll, abscisic acid, and the variety of enzymes found in plants work, and how they work, we do know many of the ways these substances can help humans and animals. Some of the general findings will be presented in this chapter, including evidence of the remarkable blood cleansing and building abilities of chlorophyll, its effect on the circulatory system and oxygen supply, and its role in detoxifying and regenerating the liver. I will also discuss its use as a body deodorant. Chapters 6 and 8 will discuss how wheatgrass affects specific ailments.

GUARDING AGAINST
ENVIRONMENTAL HAZARDS

With such a great emphasis placed on cleanliness in our society, it's a wonder so few people are concerned about the problem of internal filth. After years of living in polluted surroundings we shouldn't be so naive as to believe that we have eliminated efficiently and perfectly every toxin we have consumed via the food we eat, air we breathe, and water we drink. In reality, not one person alive is unaffected by environmental hazards.

Air currents carry toxic levels of lead, cadmium, and carbon monoxide, which affect our liver, lungs, and metabolic functions. Our water supply is contaminated with chlorine bleach and sodium fluoride, which can cause headaches and nausea. The food we purchase in supermarkets contains chemical additives such as nitrates, monosodium glutamate, Nutrasweet (aspartame), bleaching agents, and synthetic antioxidants like BHT and BHA—all of which can cause allergic reactions and place an excessive strain on the liver and excretory organs.

Only recently have the contaminants in our air, food, and water been tested to see exactly what harm they do us. The results are grim. Some of them are carcinogenic (cancer-causing) or mutagenic (capable of altering genes or DNA, and possibly affecting future generations). Since we can't really avoid all of these things in our environment all of the time the best we can hope to do is strengthen our bodies so we can co-exist with them, and yet not be devastated by them.

Chlorophyll can protect us from carcinogens like no other food or medicine can. It acts to strengthen the cells, detoxify the liver and bloodstream, and chemically neutralize the polluting elements themselves.

Japanse scientists working along with Yoshihide Hagiwara, M.D., found that the enzymes and amino acids in young grass plants deactivated the carcinogenic and mutagenic effects of 3,4 benzpyrene, a substance found in smoked fish and charcoal-broiled meats. The enzymes in grasses have also been shown to neutralize the toxicity of various nitrogen compounds found in automobile exhuast. According to Tsuneo Kada, director of the Japan Research Center of Genetics, these tests show that grasses have a wider range of metabolic activity than animals and humans, and are capable of more efficient neutralization and detoxification of certain pollutants. It has been my experience that by including wheatgrass juice in the diet, we can protect ourselves from pollution. The enzymes that seem to be particularly effective in strengthening the body's defenses are superoxide dismutase (SOD), protease, amylase, and catalase.

A recent experiment by Dr. Chiu-Nan Lai at the University of Texas points in the same direction. Dr. Lai showed that wheatgrass juice had a powerful anti-mutagenic effect. In addition, it showed anti-neoplastic ability (the ability to fight tumors) without the usual toxicity of drugs that also inhibit cell-destroying agents.

WHEATGRASS ENZYMES: TOP-NOTCH BLOOD CLEANSERS

The many active compounds found in grass juice can cleanse the blood and neutralize and digest toxins in our cells.

I like to think of the human body as a gigantic biologically active chemical factory. Under the skin, millions of chemical actions and reactions take place all the time. The force behind many of these delicate metabolic operations is enzymes. Long considered catalysts (substances that affect the rate of chemical reactions, but are not changed by them), enzymes are now understood by many scientists to be more than mere supplementary material; they are life energy itself. Whether you want a cut on your finger to heal or you desire to lose five pounds, enzymes must be called upon to do the actual work. In fact, every action from thinking to digesting food or moving your legs requires the activity of thousands of enzymes. Enzymes are especially vital to the process of blood cleansing.

We can employ two basic types of enzymes in the process of cleansing and rebuilding our blood, and, ultimately, our bodies. The first group is *indogenous enzymes*, which are found inside us. While this group is powerful and capable of great detoxification, indogenous enzymes do wear out with age. Their lifespan and abilities can be extended if we help them from the outside by adding *exogenous enzymes*, like the ones found in wheatgrass juice, to our diet.

We can only get the benefits of the many enzymes found in grass by eating it uncooked. Cooking destroys 100 percent of the enzymes in food. A certain amount of enzyme activity is also lost by prolonged exposure to air, processing, or drying. This is why I recommend that you grow your own wheatgrass and drink it within minutes of juicing.

In addition to enzymes, wheatgrass also contains amino acid chains (polypeptides) and bioflavonoids (compounds related to vitamins) that also help cleanse the blood and other tissues. The amino acids are absorbed directly into the blood. As well as neutralizing toxic substances like cadmium, nicotine, strontium, mercury, and polyvinyl chloride, by changing them into insoluble salts which the body can eliminate more easily, they stimulate cellular metabolism. The flavonoids act to detoxify cells and prevent their deterioration.

HOW WHEATGRASS BUILDS BLOOD AND STIMULATES HEALTHY CIRCULATION

Wheatgrass juice contains liquid oxygen. Oxygen is vital to many body processes: it stimulates digestion (the oxidation of food), clearer thinking (the brain utilizes 25 percent of the bodily oxygen supply), and protective oxygenation of the blood (a defense against anaerobic bacteria). It also promotes better circulation of the blood, ultimately nourishing every cell in the body.

In a conversation I had with Dr. Arthur Robinson, co-founder of the Linus Pauling Institute, he mentioned that it seems wheatgrass juice has a dilating effect on the blood vessels themselves. That is, it makes the blood vessels larger so that blood can flow through them more easily. Increased circulation means better nutrition to the cells and more efficient removal of waste from them as well; both processes are important in terms of healing or rebuilding the body. Dr. Otto Warburg, a German biochemist, won a Nobel prize for his study which revealed that cancer cells cannot exist in the presence of oxygen. Therefore, he surmised that any cancer therapy, if it were to work, would have to increase the oxygen content of the blood, especially at the site of the cancer. We will talk more about wheatgrass and cancer later.

Numerous experiments on animal and human subjects have shown chlorophyll to be effective in treating anemia (a low serum iron count). As many as 30 percent of all women beyond the age of puberty in the United States may be anemic. For men the rate of anemia begins to increase at the age of fifty. The major symptoms of anemia are fatigue and loss of appetite.

To produce healthy, iron-rich blood, key vitamins like B_{12} and folic acid, minerals like iron, copper, and potassium, and protein must all be present in adequate amounts in the diet. It is next to impossible, however, to obtain all of these from meals comprised of white bread or white potatoes, broiled meats, canned vegetables, and processed foods. While these items may contain minimal amounts of essential nutrients, processing and cooking destroys them or renders some of them non-absorbable. Since wheatgrass is always used raw, it is a good source of all the nutrients mentioned above—in a form in which they can be readily converted by the body into healthy red blood cells. The more red blood cells, the more iron-rich the blood will be.

As the Hughs and Latner study I referred to earlier pointed out, chlorophyll extracted from green plants has shown the ability to increase the hemoglobin count in experimental animals in a short period of time (see page 10). Years ago, it was commonly given to patients with iron deficiencies and proved to be effective in restoring the blood to normal.

WHEATGRASS AND LIVER FUNCTION

Another benefit of chlorophyll is the stimulation and regeneration of the liver—the main organ of detoxification in the body. The liver is the real workhorse of the body, performing more than five hundred different functions, from digestion and storage to cleansing the blood and reorganizing nutrients. Unfortunately, 90 percent of our liver function can be destroyed before any serious symptoms arise, and at that point it can be too late to correct the problem. Since the liver is responsible for removing toxic substances from our blood, when it is damaged by fatty degeneration, infectious microbes or other irritants, it weakens our blood cleansing abilities.

Three compounds found abundantly in wheatgrass help the liver stay vital and healthy. Choline works to prevent the deposition of fat, magnesium helps draw out excess fat in the same way magnesium sulfate (epsom salts) will draw pus from an infection, and potassium acts as an invigorator and stimulant.

Dr. Wattenburg of the University of Minnesota School of Medicine found that when rats were fed a diet containing all the known vitamins and nutrients, but highly purified (our modern diet is 50–75 percent purified), they were unable to manufacture certain enzymes which deactivate carcinogens in the liver. However, when the same rats were fed a portion of greens, they were able to produce the enzyme. The compound in the greens that made this possible is called an *indole*, and is found in wheatgrass.

Another interesting finding on the ability of grasses to invigorate the liver was reported by Dr. Charles Schnabel in an article called "Grass: the Forgiveness of Nature," published in *Acres USA*, in January, 1980. Writing on the nutritional and health benefits of young grasses, including wheatgrass, on both humans and animals, Dr. Schnabel compared the overall health of a flock of Leghorn hens receiving 5 percent fresh young grass in their diet to that of another flock of Leghorns being fed identical rations, with the exception of receiving alfalfa instead of grass. The grass-fed hens were far healthier than the others, as indicated by their richer, darker blood and livers (the grass-fed hens had dark mahogany-colored livers, while the alfalfa-fed hen's livers were light tan in color).

Unfortunately, not enough research has been performed on human livers, but there is good reason to believe that the addition of grass to the diet stimulates liver function and enriches the red blood cell count. The tests made by Dr. Thelma Arthur, mentioned in the Preface, also indicate the blood cleansing effect of wheatgrass in humans. At the Hippocrates Institute, guests are instructed to use wheatgrass implants, which involve putting several ounces of fresh wheatgrass juice into the lower bowel and retaining it for about twenty minutes. A portion of the juice is absorbed directly into the portal circulation, which leads to the liver. This method allows the individual to get more chlorophyll directly to the liver than he or she could comfortably drink at once. We will discuss the uses and benefits of wheatgrass implants in more detail later.

DEODORIZING PROPERTIES OF CHLOROPHYLL

One obvious way of testing the effect of wheatgrass on body toxins is the absence of foul body odors reported by users. In a study by R.W. Young and J.S. Beregi, reported in the *Journal of the American Geriatric Society* in 1980, sixty-two nursing home patients were given chlorophyll in tablet form. Although tablets are less potent than juice, they were nevertheless found to be helpful in controlling body and fecal odors. The chlorophyll also eased the severity of chronic constipation and reduced the presence of gas.

In 1950, Dr. Howard Westcott found that one hundred milligrams of chlorophyll are as good a deodorant as any other. Whereas most deodorants merely cover up a bad odor, he discovered that chlorophyll extracts successfully neutralized offensive odors in foods, alcohol, and tobacco *in vitro* (in a test tube). Moreover, in patients and volunteers, it effectively neutralized bad breath, body odor from perspiration, menstrual odors, and foul-smelling urine and stools.

In their book *Medicine Of Chlorophyll*, Drs. Keiichi Morishita and Kaneo Hotta, Japanese scientists who have studied the properties of chlorophyll for years, report that they were able to observe its remarkable deodorant properties. In one test, ten volunteers were given garlic to eat, followed by three to twelve grams of chlorophyll. In twenty minutes, the odor of garlic was not present in eight of the volunteers. The same phenomenon occurred after experimental subjects drank alcohol and smoked cigarettes. Body odor, being a secretion from inside the body that begins to smell offensive after it reacts with bacteria on the skin, is a little more difficult to correct. However, in a matter of weeks the secretions that cause the odor can be neutralized.

Scientists have known about the deodorizing properties of chlorophyll for some time. It is for this reason some drugs, chewing gum, breath fresheners, vaginal douches, and antiseptics contain chlorophyll.

The enzymes, amino acids, and chlorophyll in wheatgrass juice contain anti-bacterial compounds that are especially good at destroying anaerobic bacteria that thrive in oxygen-poor blood and tissue. Certain infections, ulcers, and putrefaction are caused in part by anaerobic bacteria that cannot live in the presence of oxygen or oxygen-producing agents such as chlorophyll. Wheatgrass juice deactivates these anaerobic bacteria and promotes regeneration of the damaged area. Yet it doesn't sting like some antiseptics, and produces no known side effects or allergic reactions.

All of the enzymatic activity in wheatgrass adds up to one vitally important thing—greater strength and resistance to pollutants both outside and inside the body.

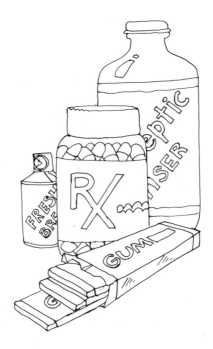

Everyday Products Containing Chlorophyllin

4

Life Extension and Rejuvenation Through Wheatgrass

... Give me a field where the unmow'd grass grows, the good green grass, that delicate miracle, the ever-recurring grass ...

Walt Whitman

As in the days of Ponce de Leon, humans everywhere are still in hot pursuit of the fountain of eternal youth. One drink from this magic fountain, it was believed, would restore youthful appearance, outlook, and vigor. Despite the fact that scientists have now discovered over a hundred chemical elements and thousands of factors that play a role in nutrition and health, they are not even one step closer to realizing the dream of eternal youth than Ponce de Leon was five hundred years ago. In fact, when you consider the rising incidence of degenerative disease in our society, you could say we have taken a few steps in the opposite direction. Yet, in wheatgrass, I believe we have a veritable fountain of youth available to us.

Many of the wild claims being made about vitamin-mineral supplements are exaggerated and misleading. Supplements, "youth drugs," or hormones will not, in any amount, cure the common cold, restore potency to an octogenarian, or return hair to a bald head. In most cases supplements are a waste of time and money, and they can even be dangerous in large doses.

Let's be clear: synthetic vitamin-mineral supplements can have a druglike effect, creating symptoms from constipation and headaches to kidney and liver damage. Furthermore, they have a limited effect compared to their natural counterparts found in fresh foods. Synthetic Vitamin E, for example, is less than one-tenth as effective as natural E. Less of the synthetic vitamins and minerals get absorbed than the forms found naturally in foods. All vitamins and minerals found in nature come "packaged" with other nutrients to ensure their optimal absorption and use. This is the way we have been getting our vitamins for millions of years—and it is still the safest and best way to do so.

Wheatgrass contains a full spectrum of vitamins and minerals, including the thirteen essential ones, packaged with dozens of trace elements and enzymes. It is a nutritionally complete food which will sustain the growth and development of laboratory animals and humans alike. In addition, scientists have never found wheatgrass to be toxic in any amount when given to either animals or humans. I will discuss the role of vitamins in nutrition more fully in the following chapter.

NUTRITION AND REJUVENATION

Proper nutrition is inseparable from the process of rejuvenation. No other method or treatment can bring assured results as quickly and permanently with total safety. Despite huge medical gains over the past one hundred years, medical solutions to life extension and rejuvenation have all fallen short— the average male lives just four years longer today than his ancestor did a hundred years ago. And until we can prevent ourselves from falling into the grave in the first place it is doubtful whether we will find a way to raise ourselves out of it.

The most sane and direct approach we have towards finding the fountain of youth is through proper nutrition, utilizing potent foods like wheatgrass and sprouts, and moderate exercise. Unfortunately, this approach requires effort, and is not as glamorous as taking an elixir—but the results more than justify the means.

My own experience exemplifies the miraculous ability of wheatgrass to fill deficiencies in the body and reverse the aging process. At fifty years of age I was ready for an early retirement. My hair was gray, I had a terrible case of colitis and other colon problems, I suffered from low energy, and had no clear direction in life. Out of desperation I turned to nature for relief. Lessons I had learned in childhood from my grandmother were strong in my memory and dreams.

My intuition and reason led me to experiment with the most vital and nutritionally rich foods I could find. These were not meats, cheeses, and eggs, as most people suspected at that time, but those foods which could trap the sun's energy and transfer it to my body. These were *live* foods—foods richer in vitamins, minerals, and life energy, than in proteins or fats. While proteins and fats are necessary, I knew that I did not need them in the heavy form and large quantities used by the average person.

I knew that to find the energy of life and use it to rejuvenate my tired and sickly body I would have to find it in green plants. Charles Kettering and a handful of other researchers had the right idea, but commercial pressures forced them to seek ways to package or synthesize the life energy in green plants to increase its shelf life—which cannot be done.

In wheatgrass, raw foods, and exercise, I found what I feel is as close to the fountain of youth as we are going to get. Twenty-five years after my discovery, my hair has turned fully natural brown again. My weight has been a stable 119 (the same as it was in my youth), and my energy level is limitless. For the past ten years I have required an average of only four hours of sleep a night, and I haven't needed the services of a physician in years. My work has brought me all over the world on many demanding lecture tours, sometimes for months at a time. Yet I have more energy than I ever remember having as a child—and I am no child at seventy-six. What I found can help you, too. But instead of taking my word for it, examine what I have to say carefully, and then, if you are so inclined, try it for yourself.

LONGER LIFE

I am not going to promise that wheatgrass will give you immortality, but it can cleanse your blood and help rejuvenate aging cells, slowing the aging process down, way down, making you feel more alive now. Americans as a group do not live long. In many areas, such as personal income and production, we lead most other nations year after year, but when it comes to longevity, in 1978 we ranked about twenty-fifth for men and ninth for women. American men live an average of sixty-nine years and women seventy-four. People in Israel, Greece, Japan, East Germany, and Australia live longer than we do. Women in the Netherlands, Iceland, Sweden, Norway, Denmark, France, Canada, and Britain all live longer than American women.

Compared to our American ancestors, however, we are doing better. Of course they had to deal with pestilence, famine, and more infant and maternal deaths. Just the same, in 1900 the average life expectancy in America was forty-seven, and by 1950 it had risen by twenty years. In the three decades since then any increase in lifespan has been insignificant. The problem is that we have changed our diet radically. The average American now consumes about nine pounds of chemical additives per year. Nearly 50 percent of the food in the typical American diet is artificially processed. Americans eat fewer fresh vegetables and fruits and more red meats, poultry, and dairy products, than ever before.

There are no deep secrets to living a long life. Simplicity is the key. That is what we can learn from the traditionally longevinous peoples of Hunza, Pakistan; Vilcabamba, Equador; and Georgia, Russia. A simple diet that includes plenty of chlorophyll-rich greens, fresh vegetables, sprouted grains, beans, seeds, fresh fruits, and other wholesome foods, with few (if any) animal foods, is best. The addition of wheatgrass to such simple fare creates a diet with the power to regenerate the body far better than any chemicals, drugs, or vitamin-mineral supplements can.

Think about it for a moment. Can you get life from non-living things? If you plant a vitamin pill in the ground, will it sprout up and grow into a thick living plant? Of course not. How then can it add life and energy to your body in the same way that living wheatgrass, greens, or sprouts can? Plant any of these in the ground and they will create new life out of the soil, rain, and air. Vitamin supplements may be necessary on a temporary basis, to balance an existing problem, but they cannot take the place of live foods in the diet.

It is the life force in wheatgrass, along with its stores of vital nutrients, that can restore youthfulness to the body. If you cook the grass, what is left? A mere shell of matter, totally devoid of life. When we cook food, we destroy its enzymes and life energy. It is no small wonder that we age quickly, degenerate, and die younger than we have to.

Life comes from life. Wheatgrass, as it grows on a tray of soil in your home, is the essence of life and vitality. Wheatgrass contains extraordinary nutrients, identified by G.O. Kohler as the "grass juice factor," which he found only in grasses. The research of Kohler and others has indicated that the grass juice factor can correct nutritional deficiencies, stimulate growth, and prevent early death in herbivorous (plant-eating) animals.

Now let us briefly discuss the nutritional factors in wheatgrass chlorophyll which give the juice the ability to rejuvenate even the most tired and worn out body.

WHEATGRASS, ENZYMES, AND AGING

Enzymes are perhaps more important than any other active ingredients in wheatgrass. To date, literally hundreds of enzymes have been discovered in cereal grasses. An even more thorough study in the future may turn up thousands, because grass is a storehouse of enzymes.

When included in the diet, these enzymes supplement the indogenous enzymes manufactured in the human body (see page 19), extending their life energy. The most important enzymes that have been isolated in wheatgrass are: cytochrome oxidase, an antioxidant required for proper cell respiration; lipase, a fat-splitting enzyme; protease, a protein digestant; amylase, which facilitates starch digestion; catalase, which catalyzes the decomposition of hydrogen peroxide into water and oxygen in the blood and body tissues; peroxidase, which has an action similar to catalase, on a cellular level; transhydrogenase, an enzyme which aids in keeping the muscle tissue of the heart toned; and superoxide dismutase (SOD).

It is interesting to note that when these enzymes decline in quantity and strength—which happens as we get older—the body's ability to handle heavy fats, proteins, and excess calories weakens. This could be responsible for the problems of overweight and premature aging, which plague so many Americans today. It is also interesting to note that three of these enzymes—cytochrome oxidase, peroxidase, and catalase—are found in relatively high concentrations in normal red and white blood cells. In the body of a cancer patient, however, their numbers are usually decreased significantly.

We have already seen how the enzymes found in wheatgrass help to detoxify the pollutants inside us. They also help us to digest our food better. In some cases they also have shown an ability to "digest" or dissolve excesses of fat and protein in the body, and may even break down tumors and cysts.

One of the enzymes found in cereal grasses, SOD, plays a crucial role in wheatgrass's ability to prevent aging. This enzyme has received plenty of attention in scientific circles as a possible anti-aging enzyme.

Working independently, Dr. Barry Halliwell, a biochemist at the University of London, Dr. M. Rister, at the University of Cologne in Germany, and Dr. Irwin Fridovich, a biochemist at Duke University, have found SOD in all body cells. They have investigated the role that this enzyme plays in slowing cellular aging. Remarkably, SOD lessens the effects of radiation, acts as an anti-inflammatory compound, and may prevent cellular damage following heart attacks or exposure to irritants. Wheatgrass is a superior food source of SOD.

SOD occurs naturally in each cell as a balancing agent that neutralizes the toxic effects of superoxides, which also reside in cells. Superoxides are substances produced by every cell in the normal metabolic processes. However, when the quantity of superoxides in the cells increases without a corresponding increase in SOD production, they can damage cells and stimulate aging.

After exposure to radiation or pollutants such as nitrogen oxide derivatives, following the consumption of foreign (and toxic) substances like drugs and chemical additives, and as we age, the number of harmful superoxides in and around our cells increases. Their accumulation damages the fats, DNA, and overall structure of the cells. As I mentioned, some amount of superoxides is necessary, but any excesses should be destroyed by SOD present in cells. When the supply of SOD is low, cells become poisoned; they lose their ability to renew themselves, and die prematurely. In fact, the older or more abnormal the cells in the body, the greater the number of superoxides they usually contain.

In both laboratory trials and clinical tests, however, SOD has proven to be a safe and effective enzyme which can protect us from cell damage due to superoxides, infection, aging, radiation, and poisoning by bad food, air, or drugs. And wheatgrass is a natural source of this enzyme.

WHEATGRASS AND DNA REPAIR

Dr. Yasuo Hotta, a biologist at the University of California at San Diego, has isolated another compound from young grasses. Provisionally named P4D1, this substance has shown the ability to stimulate the production and natural repair of human reproductive sperm cells and DNA.

Dr. Hotta tested reproductive cells rather than somatic cells (the ones that make up body tissues) because of their remarkable ability to repair damaged DNA, thus ensuring the health of the newborn. The experiment consisted of first damaging one group of spermatocytes with X-radiation and administering a toxic chemical to another group. Some of the damaged cells from each group were then allowed to recover on their own, and others were given P4D1. When the cells were incubated under normal controlled conditions, the added extract increased the number of cells repaired and the speed at which the repairs took place. When the extract was added to undamaged cells it also assisted in their normal repair processes.

What this means is that young grasses, including wheatgrass, may be able to increase potency and reproductive powers. And for those who are impotent, elderly, or ill, the return of potency is a sure sign of a stronger body and greater ability to fight disease and hold off aging. Dr. Hotta is currently testing the effect of the extract on somatic cells, which are slower to recover, to see whether they too can be benefited by it.

The regenerative effect of young spring grasses also has important implications for agriculture. Dr. Charles Schnabel showed farmers how fresh young grasses returned fertility to bulls and extended the longevity of milkers by at least five or six years. Grasses have the same regenerative and productivity-increasing effect on other farm animals, too. Today, large-scale cattle farms and many city zoos use huge machines to grow grasses indoors to feed their animals year-round. If grass can return fertility to a bull, think of what it could do for you!

WHEATGRASS AGAINST FREE RADICALS

We are not leaving the subject of rejuvenation to venture off into the political arena when we discuss "free radicals." Free radicals are atoms with a bunch of wild electrons that can surround your cells internally and age every part of your body from the inside out. They are created especially by the processed and cooked fats in our diet.

A recent book by Durk Pearson and Sandy Shaw, entitled *Life Extension,* has brought much attention to free radicals. The authors point out the damage free radicals can cause, and suggest ways to eliminate them as a means to a longer and healthier life. Unfortunately, their advice could be harmful, since the drugs and supplements they recommend have not been thoroughly tested for long-term effects. Their premise is that certain chemicals called *antioxidants,* contained in food additives like BHT and BHA, can neutralize and reverse the accumulation of free radicals in the body, improving health and extending longevity.

However, according to Dr. Jeffrey Bland, a biochemist at the University of Puget Sound in Washington, preliminary results of studies on the long-term use of BHT and BHA as anti-aging supplements indicate that these food additives tend to inhibit the production, in the liver, of certain enzymes that are necessary for health and long life.

My own feeling is that the practice of using preservatives to extend lifespan is absurd. Preserving a food item and preserving the life of a living body by using food additives are galaxies apart. Do you want to be preserved while you're still alive? I don't! While portions of the cell have a vital need for oxygen, other parts may be damaged by it. Antioxidants protect these important components of the cell (especially unsaturated fats) from being damaged by oxygen. The antioxidants found in BHT, BHA, and other additives are also found in wheatgrass and other natural foods, in a form which is both safer and more efficient than the chemical types.

As you may recall, I have mentioned that fats can accumulate as certain enzymes diminish due to age and poor eating habits. What I didn't discuss was *how* these fats contribute to premature aging and how wheatgrass can remove them, and that is where free radicals enter the picture.

Over the past few years, many Americans have switched from saturated fats (mostly animal fats) to unsaturated and polyunsaturated ones. The unsaturated fats were supposed to prevent heart disease while the saturated fats caused it. However, now we know we were wrong. Both types of fats increase our risk of heart disease, and worse, accelerate the aging process—saturated fats by their tendency to shut off oxygen to our cells, and polyunsaturated fats for the same reason—but also because they create free radicals.

Free radicals are atoms that contain electrons which have become detached from their paired mates. In the bloodstream, they form easily from polyunsaturated fats in the presence of oxygen. They can also form outside the body in oil when it becomes rancid. The problem is that free radicals are very unstable. They tend to disrupt anything they get close to, and can damage nearly every system in the body.

According to P. Gordon, in "Free Radicals and the Aging Process," in *Theoretical Aspects of Aging,* published by Academic Press, when cells are damaged by free radicals, their remnants persist as intracellular accumulations called lipofuscin pigments. These further disrupt health by inhibiting the flow of oxygen into cells. The quantity of lipofuscin pigments usually increases with age, and can be regarded as an indication of the age of tissues. A high-fat diet like the one eaten by most Americans is believed by many investigators in the field of aging to be one of the primary ways to increase the quantity of lipofuscin pigments.

Wheatgrass, on the other hand, can prevent both free radicals and lipofuscin pigments from accumulating and doing their damage. Wheatgrass juice contains vitamins C, E, and carotene, natural antioxidants which protect us from free radical formation, safely and effectively. The antioxidants found in synthetic chemicals such as BHA and BHT may be able to prevent rancidity in polyunsaturated oils, but there is no proof that they can do the same inside the human body. In addition, there is no evidence that they are safe for supplemental use since we have only been exposed to small amounts of them for the last few years.

Vitamins A, C, and E are examples of natural antioxidants. Vitamin C not only prevents free radical formation, but also prevents vitamins A and E from being destroyed. Wheatgrass juice contains about as much Vitamin C per ounce as orange juice, and more than most common vegetables.

Vitamin A is not found in wheatgrass juice, or any other plant food, but its precursor, carotene, is. In fact, carotene is one of the substances that prevents oils from becoming free radicals while plants are alive. Unlike animal food sources of Vitamin A, which can cause harm in large doses, carotene has not been found to be toxic in any amount. In experiments where investigators gave animals extra carotene from food sources or in foods, they discovered that it had a major protective effect against the formation of free radicals in the animals' tissues.

Wheatgrass juice is a good source of Provitamin A (carotene). It has more carotene per pound than iceberg lettuce, tomatoes, and many other garden vegetables. Of course, besides using wheatgrass juice to prevent aging due to free radicals, you can limit the fats and oils in your diet to those found in foods. Cooking oils, butter, margarine, mayonnaise, and other "free" fats can age your body to the extent that you indulge in them and cannot rid your body of the excesses.

YOU ARE ONLY AS YOUNG AS YOUR BLOOD

A healthy body requires healthy, normal blood to stay that way. In my opinion, the healthier the blood, the greater the vitality and longer the span of life. For it is the quality of the blood which determines the strength of our bones and the firmness of our muscles. Without rich, healthy blood to carry nutrients to every cell of the body, we merely survive with our share of poor health and low energy.

According to Dr. Bernard Jensen, none of the blood builders are superior to green juices and wheatgrass. Over the years he has used them both to treat low serum iron count and toxic conditions of the blood. In his book *Chlorophyll Magic From Living Plant Life*, Dr. Jensen mentions several cases where he was able to double the red blood cell count in a matter of days merely by having patients soak in a chlorophyll-water bath. Blood values were measured, using standard laboratory techniques, before and after the baths. The blood building results occurred even more quickly when the patients drank green juices and wheatgrass regularly in addition to taking the chlorophyll baths. Blood rich in iron brings more oxygen to the cells, promoting youthfulness and preventing senility.

REJUVENATION THROUGH WHEATGRASS

While we still do not know exactly why wheatgrass rejuvenates poor-quality blood and tired bodies, we have many clues.

Years ago, Brown Langone wrote a book entitled *Make Your Cells Grow Younger*, in which he discussed the remarkable power of root auxins—substances found in the roots of all young, growing plants. He cited research experiments conducted by botanists who placed root auxins on the tip of a leaf, causing root to grow on the edge of the leaf. Langone reasoned that we could get a sort of youth auxin from eating baby greens, sprouts, and grasses. Others have proven his assumptions correct. For example, Dr. Weston Price, founder of the Price-Pottenger Nutrition Foundation, isolated a substance from the tips of young grasses which had a similar effect to that of root auxins, showing an ability to promote regeneration in damaged cells. My own research confirms these results.

Wheatgrass may be used as a tonic and rejuvenator because of its abundance of natural vitamins, minerals, trace elements, and enzymes. It is also a high-quality source of fuel, and it is highly assimilable, requiring little energy to digest. Even those with weak or failing digestion can reap the rewards of using it.

5

Super Nutrition From Wheatgrass

Next in importance to the divine profusion of water, light and air, those three great physical facts which render existence possible, may be reckoned the universal benificence of grass. It yields no fruit in Earth or air, yet should its harvest fail for a single year famine would depopulate the world.

Senator John James Ingalls
of Kansas, 1872

Live foods nutrition is super nutrition because it recognizes and appreciates the differences between raw and cooked foods and between natural and synthetic nutrients. In the conventional nutrition-school curriculum there is little room for a discussion of either the value of enzymes and life forces in foods, or the merits of live (raw) versus cooked foods. Yet the difference, when translated into health terms, is the difference between being vitally healthy and alive, and just breathing.

In this chapter I will discuss many of the ordinary nutritional components of wheatgrass and what I feel are some of its super-nutritional aspects. I will also compare its cost and effectiveness to some of the more popular "health" foods and synthetic vitamin-mineral supplements.

NUTRITIONAL GRASS ROOTS

We owe our existence to the grasses which spread over the earth fifty million years ago and made it habitable for animals and humans both. Regrettably we have all but forgotten this fact. Even though we drink milk and eat meat from animals that eat grass, we seem to take its marvellous nourishing properties for granted. Yet, if anything happened to our livestock and our food reservoirs dried up, it would be a comfort to know that wheatgrass, all by itself, could keep us alive and well.

Could we live on any of the other common vegetables, leaf crops, or weeds? Experience says no. For years it was assumed that herbivorous animals could live on any of the common green plants. Nowadays we know this isn't true. A guinea pig is herbivorous, yet it would die in less than thirteen weeks on a diet of lettuce, cabbage, or carrots, and would grow at half its normal rate on a diet of spinach. But the same guinea pig would thrive on a diet of only wheatgrass. In fact, Dr. Charles Schnabel developed a superior strain of guinea pigs in five generations on a diet solely of grass. But can wheatgrass sustain humans? I think so.

In any discussion comparing the nutritional values of a food substance like wheatgrass against the nutrients found in vitamin pills, it must be remembered that nature packages nutrients in a complex and balanced arrangement, whereas chemists, try as they will to duplicate nature's way, cannot. The nutrients in wheatgrass and raw foods are more readily used by the body, so that a much smaller quantity of them is required, compared to when vitamin-mineral supplements are used.

In addition, when I discuss the nutritional value of wheatgrass here, I am speaking of the liquid. When wheatgrass juice is dried, some of its nutrient values increase by a factor of twenty or more, due to the absence of water. If we were comparing wheatgrass with spirulina or chlorella, which are both dried algae products, we would need to compare wheatgrass juice in its dried form to get a fair comparison. I am not saying that dried wheatgrass juice is better—*it's* *not*—but that without the liquid, certain nutrients are more concentrated. Unfortunately, the drying process destroys some enzymes and life forces—one reason why I recommend using fresh wheatgrass in juice form at its peak of nutritional value. Another reason to use fresh juice instead of the dried form is that its Vitamin C, and certain other vitamins, are lost rapidly after it is juiced or juiced and then dried.

THE BEST KIND OF VITAMINS

Your need for vitamins varies depending on your body, occupation, and style of living. It is safe to say, however, that all of us need to get enough of certain vitamins to be healthy. There is much confusion over our needs for vitamins such as C, B-complex, A, and E, and their uses by the body. Vitamin manufacturers in their advertising campaigns give us the impression that vitamins by themselves increase energy and ward off the common cold. In fact, vitamins do not increase energy levels or make us feel better directly, but through their ability to make carbohydrates, proteins, and fats in foods available for use as energy and as "building blocks." By themselves, vitamins cannot cure disease, restore potency, or sustain life. We also need the above-mentioned food factors, which we use for energy and rebuilding our cells. While getting enough of the right kinds of vitamins is essential to good health, our need for them is minimal compared to our need for carbohydrates, proteins, and fats.

Vitamin pills are being swallowed up by Americans to the tune of more than two billion dollars per year. Yet, there is still much debate about whether these synthetic substitutes can replace the real vitamins found in foods—and whether they should. Critics warn that the uninformed who use vitamins do so at their own peril. They cite various cases of overdose and vitamin toxicity. It is clear that vitamins should be treated as drugs. Though many of them are claimed to be non-toxic, their use should be monitored carefully, as their long-term effects are still largely unknown.

On the other hand, we do know that the vitamins found in foods are completely safe and capable of sustaining one in good health. Natural foods supplied our ancestors with all the essential vitamins for millions of years. It is my feeling that while synthetics seem to work in the short run, they may have damaging side effects (in the same way that most synthetic drugs do).

In addition, some people use a daily vitamin supplement to take the place of proper nutrition, often replacing the very foods that are rich in vitamins. Unfortunately, there is no guarantee that anyone can remain healthy on vitamin pills and fast foods. In fact, from what we do know such a lifestyle will most likely end in chronic illness and premature death.

The superstitious belief in abiogenesis, the theory of the production of living from non-living matter, has led many of us to the illogical conclusion that synthetic foods and supplements can not only keep us healthy, but can regenerate the body and extend its lifespan. I believe in biogenesis, the doctrine that living things are produced only from living things—and my years of experience in the field of natural health bolster my opinion. Simply put, living bodies need some live (raw) foods: that is the law of nature.

There is really no substitute for the vitamins found in high-quality raw foods. I also recommend the use of three to six ounces of fresh wheatgrass juice every day or so as added protection from the pressures and stresses of modern living. This small amount of green juice alone will supply nearly as much vitamins and minerals as the food the average person eats each day.

WHEATGRASS VERSUS THE NEW "SUPERFOODS"

You may be resisting the use of wheatgrass on the grounds that you are already using one or another of the so-called "superfoods" available from health food stores. Few of these foods, including spirulina, bee pollen, chlorella, and dried, powdered wheatgrass, have stood the test of time.

Chlorella and spirulina, both green algae, are far from being live foods—a claim which their sellers often make. Both products are single-celled organisms that are surrounded by a durable shell. In order to obtain the nutrients that are inside, the shell must be crushed open, allowing the contents to oxidize. To limit further oxidation, the algae come packaged in lightproof containers, but damage has already been done. In addition, the algae are heat-dried at temperatures in excess of 160° degrees F, which further undermines their digestibility and nutritional value. Besides, there is no evidence that humans have used either of them as food. The reason for this may be that the algae possess genes and elements which haven't evolved since their beginnings more than three billion years ago.

Beyond these limitations, German and Japanese researchers have found that chlorella is hard to digest and productive of unwanted nucleic acids. But the biggest drawbacks of the "superfoods" are their unavailability, poorly controlled quality, and, worst of all, price. A daily supply of fresh wheatgrass juice is about one or two cents, compared to a dollar or more for the others.

Another advantage of wheatgrass juice is that it can be used at its peak of nutritional value, only seconds after it is cut and juiced. The vitamins in dried "superfoods" and in vegetables lose some of their potency as soon as they are picked or cut. The Vitamin C contained in a crushed raw tomato, for example, decreases by 50 percent in about five minutes and by up to 70 percent in twenty minutes. After cooking, even more of the Vitamin C is lost. (This is another reason why I recommend that you eat as much of your food as possible uncooked.) Although wheatgrass loses much of its vitamins and enzymes soon after it is picked, it is always used raw, and if you grow your own wheatgrass at home, you will be able to use it right away.

Being a liquid, wheatgrass juice is rapidly assimilated by the body. When you drink fresh wheatgrass juice, one of the first things that strikes you is its sweetness. This rush of flavor indicates that the juice is making direct contact with the mucous membranes in the mouth and is acting immediately on the surface of the gustatory nerves. Vegetables, on the other hand, do not possess this burst of flavor unless they are juiced, because their nutrients are locked inside their fibrous cells. Cooking, which tends to break down cellulose, releases more flavor in some vegetables, but it also destroys their enzymes and other nutrients.

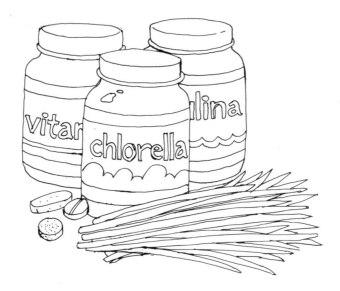

Some So-Called "Superfoods"

VITAMINS IN WHEATGRASS

Nutritionally, wheatgrass juice contains about the same amount of Vitamin C as citrus and other fruits, and more than common vegetables like tomatoes or potatoes. As you know, Vitamin C is important to the health of the skin, teeth, gums, eyes, muscles, and joints. It also aids general growth and development and acts as an antioxidant.

Wheatgrass juice supplies about as much Vitamin A as dark green varieties of lettuce (but three times more than iceberg), and more than most fruits. Dried wheatgrass juice contains as much Vitamin A as carrots, kale, or apricots, which are all high in A. Keep in mind that this is Provitamin A, also known as carotene, which is converted into Vitamin A in the intestines as needed, and is harmless in any amount. The Vitamin A found in liver, fish oils, animal foods, and most vitamin-mineral supplements accumulates in the liver and becomes toxic in large doses. Vitamin A is essential for normal growth and development, good eyesight, and reproduction. Without Vitamin A, we may suffer from weak or brittle bones, night blindness, dry skin, and lowered resistance to infection and illness. Recently, investigators have also been looking into A as a potential anti-cancer vitamin.

Wheatgrass is a good source of B vitamins, which facilitate the use of carbohydrates for energy, and aid the nervous and digestive systems. A steady supply of B vitamins is also essential for normal brain and body development, and for the adrenal glands. Our need for this anti-stress vitamin increases with the amount of physical and mental stress we encounter, though relative to the other vitamins mentioned, our need for the B complex is small.

Vitamin E, an antioxidant and fertility vitamin, is also found in wheatgrass. Without enough of this fat-soluble vitamin, we face muscle degeneration, sterility, and slower healing of wounds and infections. Vitamin E is also a protector of the heart. The type of E found in wheatgrass is about ten times more easily assimilated by the body than synthetic E. Other good live food sources of Vitamin E are sprouted seeds, grains, and nuts.

MINERALS IN WHEATGRASS

The proper quantity and quality of minerals is every bit as important as vitamins in the diet. Minerals help regulate the eliminative and blood-building functions on the molecular level, through their bonds with the many enzymes in the body. Without enough of the right kinds of minerals we can easily become toxemic and run down.

Minerals are our lifeblood. Years ago, minerals in the ancient ocean mixed with amino acids and enzymes and made life forms. Mineral salts are basic to all life. Found in both plants and animals, mineral salts are responsible for the transference of electrical current through them. They are organic, as opposed to the inorganic minerals found in stone, dietary mineral supplements, or in rusty nails.

While studies have indicated that inorganic minerals can be taken into the body and will serve a specified function, you need to take about ten to twenty times more of them to get the same effect as from organic mineral salts. When the diet includes large quantities of inorganic minerals, there is a significant risk of overload. The Bantu of southern Africa, for example, have a high incidence of liver poisoning due to their exclusive use of iron pots in cooking.

To meet your body's mineral needs I recommend you get mineral salts from wheatgrass and other live foods. By doing so, you will guard yourself against deficiency, keep your bones and teeth in great shape, and protect the many delicate metabolic functions that require the proper balance of mineral salts. When using inorganic minerals, you run a greater risk of upsetting this delicate balance and reaping chaos internally. The old adage that nature is the best chemist still rings true when it comes to getting the right kind of minerals for health.

Minerals are also important in maintaining a smooth metabolism, especially in the area of blood pH (relative acidity or alkalinity of the blood). Under normal circumstances our blood maintains a slight alkalinity, having a pH between 7.3 and 7.45 (on the pH scale, below 7.0 is acid and above 7.0 is alkaline). As a result of metabolism, acids are constantly being produced. These acids must be neutralized by alkaline minerals in order to maintain healthy bones and teeth and to promote immunity from colds and more serious illnesses. Wheatgrass has an alkalizing effect on the blood, due to its abundance of alkaline minerals such as magnesium, potassium, and calcium.

Wheatgrass is a good source of calcium, which helps build strong bones and teeth and regulates heartbeat, in addition to acting as a buffer to restore balance to blood pH. Dried wheatgrass juice has about as much calcium as milk. Juices from sprouts and green leafy vegetables, sea vegetables, and sprouted seeds, beans, and grains are also good sources of calcium in a form that is easily used by the body.

I do not recommend that you use milk or dairy as regular food items because they are too rich in saturated animal fats and cholesterol. After it has been pasteurized, homogenized, and supplemented with synthetic Vitamin D, milk is difficult for the average person to digest. Thus it is essential for you to eat plenty of greens, sprouts, and sea vegetables, along with wheatgrass juice, to be assured of getting all the calcium you need. This is especially true for people suffering from arthritis, rheumatism, muscle cramps, or tingling of the extremities—all signs of calcium deficiency. Keep in mind that up to 99 percent of the calcium we eat is deposited in our bones and teeth, and calcium cannot be properly absorbed unless other trace minerals are present along with it—as is the case in wheatgrass juice and fresh, live foods.

Wheatgrass is also a fairly good source of iron, a mineral that is essential to red blood cell formation and the transport of oxygen from the lungs to the cells. Some of our iron is reused, but we still must have a steady supply of dietary iron. Without enough iron, we can easily become tired or anemic. Women may lose needed iron during menstruation. Inorganic iron is often constipating, but the iron salts in wheatgrass have no side effects. In juice form, wheatgrass contains about half as much iron as spinach or other greens that are good sources of iron. Unlike spinach, beet greens, or chard, however, wheatgrass contains little or no oxalic acid—an element in the above-mentioned foods that binds the usable calcium in the system, can leach calcium from teeth and bones, and cause kidney stones.

Another important mineral, of which wheatgrass supplies an optimum amount, is sodium. We need sodium to aid digestion and elimination, and to regulate the amount of fluid in the body, but most Americans consume way too much of it in the form of sodium chloride (table salt) and food additives such as MSG. One proof of our need for sodium is the fact that our normal blood contains five grams of sodium per pint. The total amount of calcium in our blood is only 2 percent of the sodium content, and potassium equals only 4 percent of the amount of sodium.

However, too much sodium can cause high blood pressure, stomach ulcers, and stroke. Individuals on a low-sodium or sodium-restricted diet may use wheatgrass juice as it contains relatively little sodium compared to most prepared foods. Its sodium content is about equal to what is found in an onion or tomato.

Potassium, called the youth mineral by some nutritionists, helps maintain a smooth mineral balance, and balanced body weight. It also tones the muscles, firms the skin, and promotes overall beauty. Fruits, especially bananas, are well known for their good supply of potassium. Wheatgrass juice contains about as much potassium as citrus fruits, grapes, apples or melons.

You will find about as much magnesium in wheatgrass as in broccoli, Brussels sprouts, beets, carrots, or celery. Magnesium is important for good muscle function and for bowel health, as it aids eliminative functions. I believe that this vital mineral is also responsible for drawing fat out of the liver in cases of fatty infiltration there.

Wheatgrass is also an excellent source of a wide variety of trace minerals. These minerals are important even though they are found only in "trace" amounts inside us. One of these, selenium, is being tested for anti-cancer properties, and others, like zinc, which is essential for hair growth, many liver functions, and the synthesis of protein, are now recognized as essential for plants and animals alike.

AMINO ACIDS (PROTEIN) IN WHEATGRASS

Next to water, protein is the most plentiful nutrient in the body. More than 50 percent of the dry weight of the body is protein. Proteins, in turn, are composed of smaller proteinous "chains" called amino acids. Amino acids can be compared with the raw materials used in building a house, whereas enzymes do the actual building. Together, enzymes and amino acids are responsible for cell renewal and a huge array of diverse functions from the creation of hormones to building of muscles, blood, and organs.

There are eight amino acids, called "essential" amino acids, which the body can synthesize only from the proteins we eat. If these amino acids are not present in our food, our bodies are unable to rejuvenate our cells properly and deficiency symptoms arise. In addition to these eight, there are a dozen other amino acids which are really just as essential—but can be formed by the body internally.

Amino acids are involved in so many body systems and functions that it is beyond the scope of this book to mention them all. Let's suffice to say that they are essential to proper digestion and assimilation of foods, strong immunity against disease, rapid healing of cuts and wounds, proper liver function, and regulation of our level of mental awareness. Above all, the action of amino acids on cells in the process of self-renewal rejuvenates us and prolongs life.

A deficiency of just one amino acid can result in allergies, low energy, sluggish digestion, poor resistance to infection, and premature aging. The replacement of that amino acid can as easily result in the complete reversal of these symptoms. In essence, an adequate supply of amino acids can make the difference between fair health and low energy levels, and vital health, mental clarity, and a strong resistance to germs and other microbes. I will now discuss the seventeen amino acids found in wheatgrass juice, beginning with the eight essentials.

Lysine is one amino acid that has been receiving attention lately as a potential anti-aging factor. Body growth and blood circulation are fostered by this important amino. Without enough lysine, our immune response weakens, sight may be affected, and fatigue can occur. Another essential, isoleucine, is also needed for growth, especially in infants, and for protein balance in adults. A deficiency of isoleucine could end in mental retardation, as it affects the production of other amino acids.

Leucine is an amino acid that keeps us alert and awake. In fact, it is not recommended that insomniacs use this amino by itself as it can worsen their problem. Nevertheless, an adequate supply of leucine is necessary for anyone who wants to experience high-energy living.

Another amino acid you may have heard of, or seen listed in many vitamin-mineral formulas, is tryptophane. It is essential for building rich, red blood, healthy skin, and hair. Working with the B complex vitamins, tryptophane also helps to calm the nerves and stimulate better digestion.

Other essential aminos include phenylalanine, which aids the thyroid gland in its production of thyroxin hormone—necessary for mental balance and emotional calm; threonine, which stimulates smooth digestion, assimilation of foods, and overall body metabolism; and valine, which activates the brain, aids muscle coordination, and calms the nerves. A deficiency of valine may lead to nervousness, mental fatigue, emotional outbursts, and insomnia.

The last of the eight essential amino acids is methionine, which helps cleanse and regenerate kidney and liver cells. It also may stimulate hair growth and mental calmness. Its effect is nearly opposite that of leucine; methionine calms rather than hypes the emotions and mental processes.

Briefly, some of the other amino acids in wheatgrass are: alanine, a blood builder; arginine, which is especially vital to men, since seminal fluids contain large amounts of it; aspartic acid, a helper in the conversion of food into energy; glutamic acid, which improves mental balance and provides for smooth metabolic function; glycine, a helper in the process whereby cells use oxygen to make energy; histidine, which seems to affect hearing and nervous functions; proline, which becomes glutamic acid and performs the same tasks; serine, a stimulator of the brain and nerve functions; and tyrosine, which aids the formation of hair and skin and prevents cellular aging.

SUPER NUTRITION FROM WHEATGRASS CHLOROPHYLL

Of all the valuable compounds contained in wheatgrass juice, chlorophyll is one of the most important. If it weren't for its delicate nature, I think it would be one of the top weapons in the medical arsenal. Its instability is of no concern to you or me, however, because we can grow, juice, and drink wheatgrass without having to store it for long periods. In the next chapter and in Chapter 8 I will discuss many of the applications of wheatgrass juice in healing. Here I would like to talk about the nutritional value of chlorophyll and its conversion into blood in the body.

By itself, chlorophyll, a proteinous compound found in the green leaves of plants and grasses, isn't anything special in the eyes of most nutritionists and biochemists. But there are two vital aspects of chlorophyll which should not be overlooked.

First is its role in converting the sun's energy into a form that plants (and animals and people) can use. Chlorophyll is a sort of living battery. An animal's body also stores and produces heat and energy: the difference is that plants can get their energy directly from the sun, whereas animals and humans cannot.

In essence, the same life force in nature that explodes into greenery every spring can be transferred into the human body via the consumption of wheatgrass juice. The body can then use this super-nutritious, vital energy to heal and repair itself as needed. Again, it is very important to juice the grass right after it is cut and drink the juice immediately.

The second important nutritional aspect of chlorophyll (as you may recall from our discussion in Chapter 2) is its remarkable similarity to hemoglobin, the compound that carries oxygen in the blood.

Dr. Yoshihide Hagiwara, a Japanese scientist and health educator, is a leading advocate for the use of grass as food and medicine. He reasons that since chlorophyll is soluble in fat particles, and since fat particles are absorbed directly into the blood via the lymphatic system, that chlorophyll can also be absorbed in this way. It is his opinion that inside the body the magnesium ion in chlorophyll is replaced with an iron molecule, making new blood. In other words, when the "blood" of plants is absorbed in humans it is transformed into human blood, which transports nutrients to every cell of the body.

Only time and more research into the question will resolve the mystery of why chlorophyll works as it does. But we don't have to wait to get the benefits.

6

Healing Miracles
with Wheatgrass

*In the future man will use the sunshine element of plants to
regenerate and heal the human body.*

George Crile, M.D.

Around the 1940s the use of chlorophyll in medicines, tooth-
pastes, and breath fresheners came in vogue. Leading newspa-
pers and magazines, including *Readers Digest*, ran articles on
the promise of chlorophyll in medicine and personal hygiene.
In July of 1940, a comprehensive report written by Dr. Benjamine Gurskin, director of experimental pathology at Temple
University, was published in the *American Journal of Surgery*.
For the first time, chlorophyll was singled out as an effective
and important drug. The paper was prepared by Dr. Gurskin
and two colleagues, Drs. Redpath and Davis, both ear, nose,
and throat specialists. Some 1,200 cases of patients treated
with chlorophyll were mentioned. The complaints ranged
from deep internal infections and ulcers to skin and gum
problems. Dr. Gurskin commented on his associates' experience with chlorophyll: "It is interesting to note there is not a
single case recorded in which improvement or cure has not
taken place."

Since then, other researchers have also had success in treating a variety of disorders with chlorophyll extracts. In a study
of twenty patients with colon problems, including ulcerative
colitis (the problem I suffered with for a time), rectal implants

of chlorophyll were employed as a retention enema once a day. Patients were instructed to retain the juice for up to five hours. Doctors H.A. Rafsky and C.I. Krieger reported improvement in a majority of cases, with no side effects or irritation in any of them.

Dr. Carroll Wright, professor of dermatology at Temple University in Philadelphia, employed a chlorophyll ointment in combating several types of skin diseases. He found it to be especially useful in the treatment of chronic skin ulcers and impetigo.

Dr. W.S. Morgan, also working in Philadelphia, reported using chlorophyll to treat forty patients with eleven different types of skin problems. One of the first things the patients noticed was that chlorophyll relieved itching and burning on the skin almost immediately. A number of weeks after the study began, all but six of the original forty patients were cured—some of them freed from chronic problems they had suffered with for years.

Homer Judkin, D.D.S., of the Paris Hospital in Paris, Illinois, sent shock waves through the dental community when he announced his success in controlling Vincent's angina (trench mouth) and advanced cases of pyorrhea through the injection of chlorophyll into the gums. Discussing the recovery of a group of his patients, Dr. Judkin remarked, "In less than thirty days the gums tightened up entirely, and have remained clean ever since."

But despite all the interest in chlorophyll and its successes in clinical trials during the 1940s, there seemed to be little room for its highly unstable nature in the commercial evolution of modern medicine. Though a few companies did synthesize chlorophyll, the results of its use were inconsistent.

As it turns out, "crude" or raw chlorophyll is difficult to work with and even more difficult to store. In a matter of hours after its extraction and exposure to light and air, it loses its biochemical activity and green hue. Scientists soon learned how to obtain a synthetic chlorophyll, called chlorophyllin, by decomposing natural chlorophyll and binding it with a copper ion. Chlorophyllin kept its color, and was stable enough to store indefinitely. The only trouble was that it didn't work like the real thing. In fact, the impostor gave rise to side effects like anemia and nausea. It was abandoned for medical purposes but remains on the market as an ingredient in deodorants and as a synthetic colorant.

Slowly, chlorophyll, especially wheatgrass chlorophyll, is coming back into the medical spotlight. I have made it my life's work to bring the simple truth of grasses and other healing live foods to those in need. Along the way I have been witness to thousands of people who have improved their health and their lives. I have also collected much data regarding the particular problems that chlorophyll and wheatgrass juice can help.

Now let us turn to a brief discussion of the uses of wheatgrass in some serious but common disorders. In Chapter 8, I will present more details on the internal and external applications of wheatgrass juice.

WHEATGRASS AND OVERCOMING CANCER

For many years I have taken a great interest in the problem of cancer. My reasoning has been that if wheatgrass and live foods can help the most feared and uncontrollable medical problem, cancer, no questions should remain about its ability to heal, nourish, and balance the body. With twenty years of teaching cancer patients behind me, I know that—contrary to popular belief—all types of cancer can be overcome. However, my own opinion is that we will never find a "cure" for this dreaded problem because it can't be cured. The body of the cancer patient must heal itself in the very same way any body rebounds from a cut, bruise, or common cold. Although there are drugs which seem to help by destroying this or that cancer cell, all they can do is help. The body must replace the lost cells with new cancer-free ones.

Once you understand the logic of self-healing and self-cleansing it is easy to understand how the body can reverse even a serious problem like cancer. All that is needed is sufficient will to live and fight the disease, and enough life energy in the body—a strong enough immune system. How do you build up the immune system to overcome or prevent cancer? First, by eliminating the things that reduce your immunity: stress at home or at work, and processed and cooked foods. Once you have taken some of the pressure off your immune system in this way, you must learn how to rebuild it. Thus, your second task is to cleanse the toxic residues of stress and bad food choice from your system with a cleansing live food diet and wheatgrass.

Live foods and wheatgrass juice will begin the process of cleansing and rebuilding the immune system as long as you stay clear of the stresses and foods that create a high risk of cancer in the first place. If you do not avoid stresses, you are like a person with a broken leg who continues to walk on the leg without a cast and crutches. You won't heal regardless of how calm you are or how well you eat. Until you get off the leg and rest it nothing will help. Similarly, if you don't take a vacation (I recommend a permanent one) from the foods that congest and clog your body, your chances of recovery will be that much poorer.

While wheatgrass juice helps to build immunity, its beneficial effects range much further. Preliminary studies have identified a number of substances in wheatgrass juice that are formidable anti-cancer agents. One of these is called abscisic acid. I first learned of abscisic acid from Eydie Mae Hunsberger, a former Hippocrates guest who used the Hippocrates Diet and wheatgrass juice to heal herself of malignant breast cancer. As she relates in *How I Conquered Cancer Naturally*, her doctor took an interest in her case and researched many past studies to find the active ingredient in wheatgrass that helped make her well.

What he discovered was abscisic acid, a plant hormone known to prevent seeds from germinating until environmental conditions are just right. In tests on laboratory animals, he found that even small amounts of abscisic acid proved to be "deadly against any form of cancer." Tumors disappeared quickly in animals given injections of abscisic acid. Eydie Mae did mention, however, that research with abscisic acid is in its infant stages and it is still too early to tell whether it will become a "cure." But as she says, "Poor eating habits cause

more diseases than cancer. We may be able to reverse cancer
with abscisic acid pills, but then die from a heart attack or
something else." Only sound preventive nutrition and a healthful lifestyle can save us from all illness. Eydie Mae's decision
to switch from the "condemned person's diet" to wheatgrass
and other live foods on the Hippocrates Diet certainly paid off
for her—within one year after she was given up by the medical
establishment, the cancer was in remission—and it remained
that way.

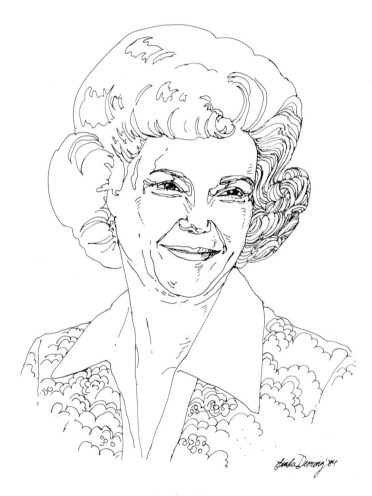

Eydie Mae

Another possible anti-cancer property of wheatgrass juice, first brought to my attention in a lecture given by the well-known biochemist and researcher, Dr. Ernst Krebs, Jr., is Vitamin B_{17} (laetrile). In his research, Dr. Krebs extracted laetrile from apricot pits, but it is also found in whole foods and especially wheatgrass. This vitamin has shown the ability to selectively destroy cancer cells, while leaving non-cancerous ones alone. While laetrile as a cancer treatment is still hotly debated in this country, the facts speak for themselves: the modern American diet contains about four hundred times less Vitamin B_{17} than the diet of the natives in countries where the incidence of cancer is extremely low.

At the Linus Pauling Institute of Science and Medicine, Dr. Arthur Robinson studied the various effects of live foods, wheatgrass, and synthetic Vitamin C on cancer in laboratory mice. Skin cancer was induced in the mice through exposure to ultraviolet radiation. The control group received the standard laboratory chow diet. Two other groups of mice were given the chow diet and different dosages of Vitamin C. Another two groups of mice received a raw foods diet restricted to apples, pears, carrots, tomatoes, sunflower seeds, bananas, and wheatgrass. One of these groups was also given one hundred grams of Vitamin C.

In a March, 1984 article entitled "Living Foods and Cancer," Dr. Robinson summarized the findings of his research as follows: "The results were spectacular. Living foods [including wheatgrass] alone decreased the incidence and severity of cancer lesions by about 75 percent. This result was better than that of any nutritional program that was tried. It was possible to duplicate this cancer suppression with ascorbic acid [Vitamin C] only by giving doses so high as to be nearly lethal for the mice and far beyond any rational range of human consumption. In fact, ascorbic acid in the amounts usually recommended for colds and cancer doubled, increased by 100 percent, the incidence and severity of the cancer."

In my own opinion, if the group of mice receiving only wheatgrass and raw foods had been given sprouts rather than fruits and vegetables, the decrease in cancer would have been even more dramatic.

The severity of cancerous lesions in Robinson's mice was caused to vary greatly by nutritional means alone. I believe that this indicates that cancer research of the future must look to diet for the answers.

The cancer-nutrition connection is becoming more evident to researchers and physicians. Recently, the prestigious National Cancer Institute commissioned the National Academy of Sciences to study the relationship between diet and cancer. The study pointed out many carcinogenic foods and their link to cancer. You may already be aware of some of them—processed items such as luncheon meats, smoked meats, high-fat cheeses, and refined oils. The study also found that some vegetables, especially green and yellow varieties, seem to have anti-cancer properties. Nevertheless, many of the foods singled out by the National Academy of Science, including carrots, squashes, broccoli, cabbage, Brussels sprouts, and leafy greens, are less potent in overall nutrition than wheatgrass—and none of them contain active enzymes when they are eaten cooked.

Oxygen Intake and Cancer

One very interesting theory offered on the problem of cancer has come from Nobel prize winner Otto Warburg, M.D., who showed that cancer cells thrived in an oxygen-poor environment. He viewed cancer not as a virus, but as a process of cell mutation caused by oxygen deprivation on the cellular level. Warburg arrived at his discovery more than fifty years ago, yet his theory still stands uncontradicted, while dozens of others are discredited every year.

We now know that things like smoking, high protein intake, air pollution, poor breathing and lack of exercise, and years of high fat consumption can starve the body of up to 25 percent of its available oxygen. According to Warburg's theory, it's no wonder that Americans suffer from one of the highest cancer rates in the world—our lifestyle, food, and environment all tend to reduce the flow of oxygen to our cells. Fresh juices, deep breathing, and wheatgrass all bring oxygen into the body, stimulating better circulation of the blood and increasing the body's oxygen carrying capacity. They also create an increase in the number of red blood cells.

We may not know the exact mechanism that helps wheatgrass juice destroy cancer cells, but we do know that in the few short years since scientists have began to look into the nutrition-cancer link they have already come up with a number of possibilities.

CAN WHEATGRASS END THE BATTLE OF THE BULGE?

Most people don't want to get fat, but few regard obesity with the panic and fear that accompany the thought of cancer. Yet there is little doubt that obesity is the biggest health problem people of western nations face today. Not because of the mental anguish fat people must face, but because being fat is not healthy. The truth of this statement is easily understood when you consider the numerous problems, including heart disease, diabetes, arthritis, high blood pressure, and cancer, which increase in both incidence and severity in people who are overweight.

Whereas excess weight used to be looked upon as a symbol of the leisure class, today it affects all sectors and age groups of our society. It does its damage quietly. At present there are more than fifty million obese people in America alone, and the problem seems to be getting worse rather than better.

Most people put on weight slowly as their metabolism fails to use or eliminate the excess nutrients they consume. The best way I know of to turn this process around is to increase the metabolic rate by becoming more physically active, by eating foods that stimulate better circulation, and by avoiding all processed foods, including sugar, red meats, dairy products, poultry, oils, and fish. Of course, using wheatgrass juice will also help, but it won't make you slim all by itself.

One of the most satisfying discoveries I have made since beginning my work in nutrition is the dramatic weight loss obtainable while using wheatgrass and following the Hippocrates Diet. The Hippocrates Diet consists of vegetables, fresh fruits, sprouts, baby greens, sea vegetables, and sprouted seeds, nuts, and grains, all eaten raw, and prepared in tasty combinations.

Since this book is about wheatgrass, though, and since I have talked about the diet for weight loss in *The Hippocrates Diet and Health Program*, I will focus this discussion on the ways in which wheatgrass is instrumental in problems of weight control.

Wheatgrass helps dieters by speeding up blood circulation and metabolic rate, and by enhancing digestive powers, thereby melting the excess fat in the body. If you take a moment to consider the many roles played by enzymes, you will realize that if you lose one pound (or gain another one) it will be because of the activity (or lack of it) of the enzymes in your food and body. In his book *Enzyme Nutrition*, enzymologist Edward Howell, M.D., mentions that measurements of the enzyme content of body fat in people weighing three hundred pounds or more revealed a deficiency of fat-splitting enzymes. Even if you are not a "heavyweight," chances are that if you want to reduce, the enzymes in wheatgrass juice and raw foods can help you.

The effectiveness of live foods and fresh juices, especially wheatgrass juice, has bankrupted many complex theories about why we become fat and how to reduce quickly. At the Hippocrates Health Institute, I have never stressed weight loss because it is as natural to wheatgrass and the living foods diet as swimming is to a duck. Nevertheless, among our guests at the Institute, the average weight loss per week is between four and fifteen pounds. I am convinced that the rich supply of enzymes in wheatgrass and live foods is the deciding factor.

At one time, obese patients were given thyroid hormones to stimulate weight loss. However, in the long run these drugs actually weaken the thyroid. If you follow my instructions for growing your own wheatgrass in soil enriched with sea kelp (see Chapter 7), and drink the juice, you will be adding an excellent source of iodine to your diet. This will have a tonic effect on the thyroid gland, and can be a tremendous aid in losing weight safely.

Common sense alone will tell you that if you eat only low-calorie, clean, and lean food you are bound to lose plenty of weight safely and quickly. In addition, the abundance of bulk in the living foods diet clears out the channels of elimination so that they operate more efficiently. The liquid content of the diet cleanses the kidneys and blood, replacing stale body fluids with naturally distilled water from vegetables, sprouts, and fruits.

Of course you don't have to change your diet completely to lose weight using wheatgrass. You can achieve a gradual weight reduction merely by taking wheatgrass juice on a regular basis while emphasizing foods that are fresh and light. The myth that bananas, avocados, and other fruits and vegetables are fattening is not based on fact. It is not these foods themselves that cause you to put on weight, but rather the way in which they are prepared (cooked and canned fruit differ from raw, fresh fruit) and what they are served with (for example—bananas with ice cream). Even foods which are not generally considered fattening, such as strawberries, can lead to weight gain if they are consumed with other food products, such as shortcake and whipped cream.

FILLING UP BUT NOT OUT

If your problem isn't overweight, but underweight, I know of no better remedy than wheatgrass juice. Many overly thin people have overactive metabolisms that don't allow them to properly assimilate the nutrients in the foods they eat. In many cases what is needed is digestive stimulation (enzymes) and relaxation.

I have seen underweight people gain two or more pounds per week after adopting the Hippocrates Diet and using wheatgrass juice. Wheatgrass will help you if you need to gain weight by clearing any accumulations of mucus from the intestinal tract, allowing more food to be absorbed, and by relaxing the nervous system. In both animal experiments and my own observations at the Institute, the addition of small quantities of wheatgrass juice to the diet stimulates balanced body weight and improved blood quality. Whether you want to shed pounds or add them, the Hippocrates Diet will fill you up—but it won't fill you out unless you need and want it to.

Perhaps the most important reason to use wheatgrass during any weight control program is its ability to fill nutritional deficiencies. As we discussed in the previous chapter, wheatgrass is a complete food, containing all the known nutrients (and probably some we don't yet know about). Using it on a daily basis while trying to reshape your body is like taking out an insurance policy against any possible deficiency that could arise. In the next two chapters I will discuss the growing methods and practical uses of wheatgrass in more detail. But before I do so I would like to talk briefly about one more use of wheatgrass as a protective measure. It can help us cope with our increasingly polluted world.

ARE YOU PROTECTED
FROM THE HAZARDS OF MODERN LIVING?

Even if you can easily avoid meats, fats, and sugar in the diet, there are other menaces to health that have been created during the past one hundred years. Here I refer mainly to pollution of our air, water, and soil; radiation poisoning from nuclear waste; television and radio waves; and emissions generated by electric and electronic appliances. Can you protect yourself from these?

As I mentioned in Chapter 3, I believe there is a way we can protect ourselves from all of these health risks—and within the past few years an increasing number of scientists and researchers have begun to agree with me. One solution, of course, is to turn to wholesome live foods and sprouts, and to use wheatgrass juice daily.

We have already discussed wheatgrass's ability to destroy harmful germs and microbes, its effectiveness as an antioxidant in preserving cells, and as a stimulant in the transport of oxygen to the cells. Pollution of all types, including lead from exhaust, sulfur oxides in industrial waste, and various gasses, tends to accumulate in the body. As an antioxidant, wheatgrass can minimize the damage that these corrosive and irritating substances have on the body, both directly and indirectly.

A few years ago I was concerned about the chemical sodium fluoride, which is commonly used as a rat poison, and was being put in our water. I asked Dr. G.H. Earp Thomas of the Bloomfield Laboratories in High Bridge, New Jersey, to do an experiment for me. He placed a small amount of wheatgrass juice in a jar of regular tap water and then tested for fluoride and other chemicals present in the water. Both of us were surprised by the results. He concluded, "Fluorine rapidly combines with calcium phosphate and other kinetic elements to lose its toxic properties, and harden teeth and bones. That is why fresh grass would act as a catalyst to speedily change the acid fluorine into a beneficial component with a positive reaction. By using wheatgrass, which is comparatively rich in calcium phosphate, it would remove any free fluoric acid and change its negative charge to an alkaline calcium phosphate fluoride combination with a positive reaction." I was amazed. Not only did wheatgrass neutralize the toxic effect of fluorine—but it converted it into an ally in maintaining healthy bones and teeth! I don't recommend that you drink tap water, though; pure spring or filtered water tastes better and is much better for you. But if you cannot obtain spring or filtered water, pour a little wheatgrass juice into regular tap water, and it will make it more healthful.

The best form of protection you can have against pollution is a stronger, healthier body. Indirectly, wheatgrass protects you from pollutants by strengthening your own body's defenses against them.

Unfortunately, it doesn't seem as if nature has programmed into the human body the ability to adapt to everything that human ingenuity can devise. Whereas we have shown a reasonable adaptation to smog and other pollution (though at an unreasonable cost in terms of poorer health) there are some things to which we seem especially vulnerable. One of these is poisoning by radiation.

For many years scientists have known that radiation from X-rays in large enough dosages can cause cancer and even death. The destructive effect of radiation is at once a boon and a thorn to the modern medical treatment of cancer. It is a boon because it destroys cancer cells, and a thorn because it also kills healthy cells and may stimulate future cancer growth. In fact, radiation is one of the many methods used to induce cancer in experimental animals.

Nuclear radiation is even more dangerous. As we are all aware, should it leak into the atmosphere slowly, or be released suddenly in an explosion, the effects on the human body would be deadly.

But even the smaller doses of radiation given off by a television set can cause illness and cancer. For this reason, Congress put into law the Radiation Control Act of 1968— which protects us from our own inventions. But this legislation only *limits* the amount of radiation given off by sets, it does not *eliminate* it. Appliances, fluorescent tube lighting, and other modern conveniences can also disrupt health by altering the electromagnetic field surrounding the body. Apart from relying on federal guidelines and industry standards, consumers really do not have a practical means of monitoring radiation levels in the home.

Knowing the threat radiation is to human health and life, scientists have been busy trying to find an antidote for it. At this very moment research is being proposed to test the protective power of wheatgrass chlorophyll against radiation. The recent interest is a result of some studies performed in the 1950s and '60s by various investigators. In one project, sponsored by the United States Army, Harry Spector, Doris Calloway, and others fed several groups of guinea pigs a standard chow diet, and then exposed them to lethal doses of radiation. All of the animals died within fifteen days. The investigators then tried introducing different foods into the diet before exposing animals to the same levels of radiation. Beets did not make any difference, but cabbage and broccoli kept more than half the animals alive longer than fifteen days. The best results were obtained by feeding the guinea pigs cabbage and broccoli before and after radiation exposure. Autopsies of the vegetable-fed animals revealed larger, healthier livers, with greater stores of Vitamin A and minimal fatty degeneration.

They also showed superior gonadal development, indicating that green vegetables can protect reproductive functions. In addition, characteristic symptoms of radiation poisoning, including malnutrition and weight loss, were delayed and reduced in severity when they did appear. J.F. Duplan, a reseacher at the Academy of Sciences in Paris, France, also found that cabbage minimized weight loss and reduced the mortality rate in X-radiated animals.

Although wheatgrass wasn't used in these tests, there is good reason to believe that it would have outperformed cabbage and broccoli as protection against radiation. One reason for this is that the positive liver and gonadal changes seen after an animal's diet is supplemented with broccoli or cabbage are, according to Dr. Schnabel, even more dramatic following supplementation with wheatgrass.

7

How To Grow and Juice Wheatgrass

All flesh is grass, and all the goodliness thereof is as the flower of the field.

Isaiah 40:6

Until now we have concentrated on the theory and philosophy behind the use of wheatgrass juice as food and medicine. In this and the next two chapters I will discuss the more practical aspects and applications of wheatgrass, including growing methods, juicing, and the wheatgrass fast.

There is nothing difficult about growing your own wheatgrass at home. At the Hippocrates Institute we have created an indoor gardening system for growing buckwheat lettuce, sunflower greens, and wheatgrass. Indoor gardening requires little time and effort—and no costly supplies. In fact, a special juicer for the purpose of juicing the wheatgrass is about the only expensive item you may want to obtain. The rest of the supplies are inexpensive and can be found locally. (If you prefer, these are also available by mail. See the Appendix.)

SETTING UP AN INDOOR GARDEN

The first step in setting up your own indoor garden system will be finding a location to plant and store the trays of wheatgrass. You will also need a place to keep seeds and topsoil or compost. Since I live on the third floor of our Boston Institute,

I both plant and store all my supplies right in my kitchen. If you live in a house you may want to set up the system in your kitchen, in your basement, in your garage, on the back porch, or in a special greenhouse area. You may also choose to break up the operations, for example, by storing soil and actually planting in the basement, setting trays in upstairs windows, and soaking seeds in jars by the kitchen sink. Whatever setup you choose, though, you will need plenty of indirect sunlight for the growing plants and a warm place to start the trays off during the winter months (65-75° F is ideal).

If the thought of bringing soil into your home bothers you, and you have no place to grow things outdoors, don't panic. Although there is no real substitute for wheatgrass grown in good soil, there are ways to grow it without soil in automatic sprouters. I use one of these to grow sprouts at home, but I still prefer to use soil to grow wheatgrass and baby greens. This is because after about five days of growth young plants begin to look for nutrients not found in the seed, but found in soil. Thus, for two to five days the plants grown in automatic sprouting machines are in need of outside nutrients that are not available. The result is wheatgrass that isn't as potent as it could be. However, if soilless growing is the only way you can foresee growing and using wheatgrass, it is far better than having none at all.

GROWING WHEATGRASS

If you use the method that I recommend, you will need to seek out some good topsoil and peat moss, or a mixture of topsoil and compost. Topsoil is the first twelve to twenty inches of dark-colored soil immediately beneath the grass on your lawn, or under the leaves covering the surface of a wooded area. If you live in a city, rather than risk being jailed for digging in the park, get some topsoil from a friend in the suburbs, or buy a few large bags from a florist or garden supply store. Peat moss is also available at these shops. Instructions for setting up a composting system begin on page 74.

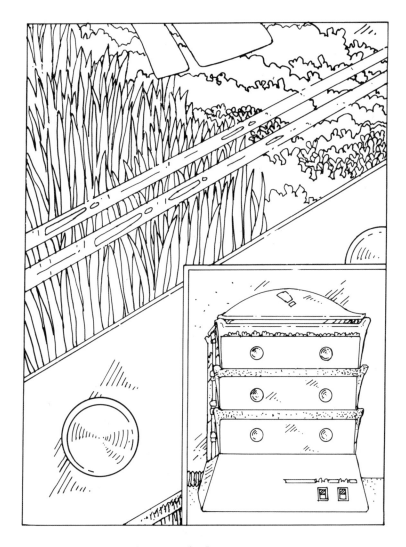

Automatic Sprouter

When taking topsoil from a wooded area, especially one where pine trees are growing, mix about a half pint of ground limestone (lime) into a trash barrel full of soil. This will offset the acidity of the soil and make your wheatgrass richer-tasting and easier to grow. Lime is inexpensive, and is available at any garden center. Ordinary lawn topsoil won't usually need lime, but you can add a handful or two per barrel full of soil just to be on the safe side. If you are using compost from an outdoor garden, it should be screened before being mixed with the topsoil, to remove large stones, sticks, and other debris. Do not use compost that has been treated with animal manures, as this may contain harmful bacteria. If you aren't mixing compost into the soil, mix soil with peat moss in a 75–25 ratio.

To produce a tray of wheatgrass per day, you will need to start off with two barrels full of topsoil and half a bale of peat moss. Along with this you will need two additional empty barrels to begin composting the used plant mats. These will take care of your soil needs for a few weeks. After that time you will be able to use the recycled soil mats from the compost barrels.

"Hard" or "winter" wheatberries are the ones we use to grow wheatgrass. These wheatberries are small, elongated grains with a deep golden color. If possible, obtain organically grown seeds from a natural foods store. Sprays and fertilizers lodged in plant fibers are toxic, and sprayed seeds do not grow well.

For planting the wheatberries I recommend that you purchase some hard plastic trays. Restaurant supply stores will often sell you cafeteria trays about 10″ × 14″ in size. Of these you will need one to hold the soil and another to cover each planted tray for the first three days of growth. So in all you will need about a dozen trays if you plan to harvest a tray per day.

To soak the wheatberries before planting, you will need some wide-mouth jars. While seeds are soaking and sprouting, cover the jars with squares of nylon mesh (available at hardware stores), and secure each with a rubber band. Try to get strong rubber bands, as weak ones can snap and the sprouts will go everywhere.

The only other things you will need are water and a little patience.

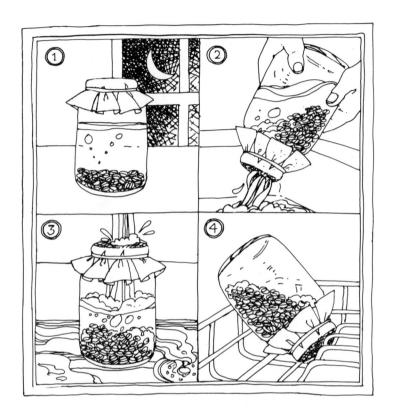

Sprouting

Planting Instructions

The amount of wheatberries to use will vary according to the size of the tray you're using, but in general one cup of dry wheatberries will be the right amount for a 10″ × 14″ tray. Before planting, wash the wheatberries to remove any grime or dust. Next, place them in a jar and fill it with water. Put a screen over the top and let it sit overnight (or for twelve hours). Drain the wheat after soaking, and rinse it well. Let it sprout in the jar at a 45° angle for another twelve hours—this makes twenty-four hours between washing the wheatberries and actually planting them.

Now spread a smooth, even layer of soil one inch deep at the bottom of the tray, leaving small trenches around the edges to catch excess water. Pour the sprouted wheat in the middle of the tray and spread it out evenly with your hands, covering the soil. Ideally, one seed should touch another on all sides, but should not have any others piled on top of it. Sprinkle the tray with water, making it damp (but not swampy), and cover with another tray.

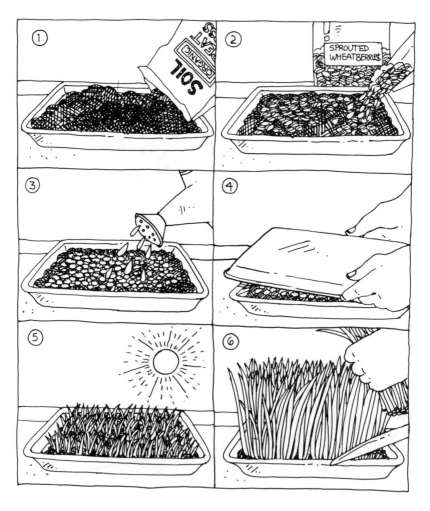

Planting

The second tray, used as a cover, creates a mini-ecosystem that duplicates the conditions under which wheat would normally grow outdoors. Beneath the cover the wheat will stay moist, warm, and protected from light, just as it would if it were covered with a thin layer of soil in the fields—but in this case the seeds stay clean and grow faster. After you have watered and covered the tray, set it aside for two to three days.

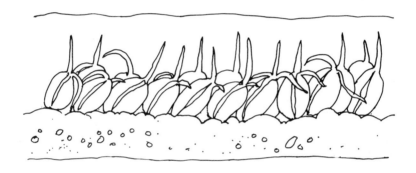

One-Day-Old Wheatgrass

At the end of two to three days (two in warmer weather and three otherwise) uncover the trays, water them, and set them out in indirect light. The two- to three-day-old wheatgrass will be about one inch high, very sturdy, and white or yellowish in color. The berry portion is barely visible at this stage. The more indirect light the plants get, the thicker and shorter the leaves and blades of grass will be, but direct sunlight will stunt their growth and dry out the soil in a couple of hours. Ideally, a balance between light and shade will produce thick, green, and juicy wheatgrass.

If you uncover a tray and see a bunch of greenish-blue mold instead of wheatgrass, you may have had bad seeds or you may have drowned them by soaking them too long. It is also possible that you over-watered the tray and/or placed it in too warm a spot to germinate. Try new seeds, less water, and a cooler location (about 65-75° F).

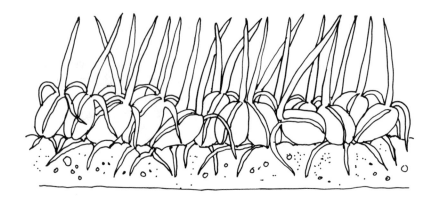

Two- to Three-Day-Old Wheatgrass

Once the trays of wheatgrass are set out in the light, they will need to be watered every day or every other day depending on the weather, humidity, and indoor temperature. The first or second time you water the plants, mix in a tablespoon of powdered kelp so that they will take up added trace minerals and iodine. Try not to muddy the soil, but keep it moist at all times. If by accident a tray is allowed to dry out, avoid the temptation to flood it with water, as this will shock the plants further. Moisten the soil instead, and make sure it doesn't dry out again for the next two days. Don't worry if the plants refuse to stand up straight again. Drooping is caused by lack of water, and the wheatgrass will still be good to eat.

After about six to twelve days your wheatgrass will be about 7–10 inches tall and ready to harvest. In cooler weather, it may take a few days longer for wheatgrass to mature fully, but during hot weather it can reach 10 inches in five days.

To harvest wheatgrass, cut as close to the soil as possible, because many nutrients are concentrated close to the soil mat. If you pull up some soil with the plants, merely rinse the root ends with plain water before juicing or eating the wheatgrass. Do not rinse the grass if you are going to store it in the refrigerator, however, as the water speeds its decomposition.

Ideally, wheatgrass should be juiced and used immediately after cutting. Although the cut grass can be stored for up to seven days in plastic bags in the refrigerator, once juiced it will begin to go bad in a half hour, and be completely spoiled in twelve hours. If wheatgrass juice is not used right away, it should be discarded.

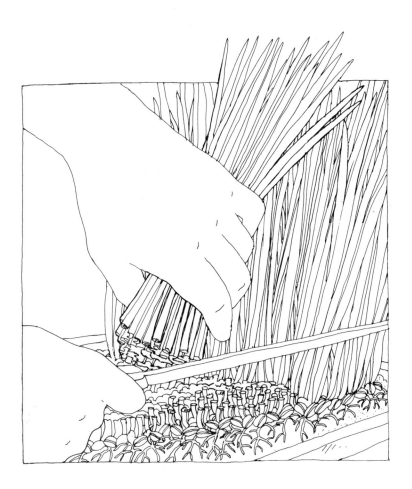

Harvesting

Planting Instructions Check List

As a handy reference guide to growing wheatgrass indoors, I have summarized the steps that we have just discussed.

- Mix 2 barrels of topsoil 50–50 with peat moss or screened compost. Obtain about 12 hard plastic cafeteria trays, several wide-mouth jars, and wheatberries to plant.

- Wash wheatberries and let them soak for 12 hours; then allow them to sprout for 12 hours.

- Spread soil 1 inch deep on trays, leaving shallow trenches around the edges to catch excess water. Smooth the soil and spread the sprouted wheatberries on top.

- Water the planted tray, cover with another tray, and set aside for 2–3 days.

- On Day 4, uncover the tray, water it, and set it in indirect light. Continue watering the tray daily or every other day, as needed, to keep it moist.

- Harvest wheatgrass with a sharp knife when it reaches 7–10 inches in height, cutting as close to the roots as possible without pulling up lumps of soil. Use wheatgrass as soon after harvesting as possible. If necessary, cut wheatgrass can be stored for up to 7 days in a covered container or plastic bag in the refrigerator.

COMPOSTING USED WHEATGRASS MATS

After you have harvested wheatgrass from the trays once or twice (it will come up several times as long as it is cut before it reaches the first jointing stage—about seven inches tall), you will be left with a mat of roots and soil that can easily be recycled into compost.

Composting is nature's way of building, improving, and maintaining the fertility of soil. In the forest, fallen leaves and dead branches cover the earth, making rich compost for the trees that continue to grow. In fact, everything that has been taken from the soil to nourish growing plants must be returned to it through decomposition of plant and animal matter if it is to continue to support new growth. Compost is a mixture of ordinary soil and plant residues that have been broken down into a rich humus by the microorganisms and worms in the soil.

The modern growing techniques used by agribusiness farmers often neglect to replace trace elements and organic material that crops take out of the soil as they grow. What little is put back most often comes in the form of synthetic chemical fertilizers. After a tract of land has been farmed in this way for a few years, its topsoil is depleted and it becomes a useless desert, barely able to sustain weeds. Acres upon acres of land all over the world are being ruined in this way every year.

Composting will prevent the problem of soil depletion in your indoor garden. It is a way of restoring natural balance. It adds organic matter and enables soil enzymes and organisms like the friendly earthworm to thrive and multiply, enriching the soil and providing the plants grown on it with top-quality nutrients. This is precisely the way nature has preserved plant life on earth for centuries. On a large scale, it is the only way we can ensure that the soil will be fertile enough to produce food for our children—and theirs.

An important worker in your compost pile is the earthworm, whose job it is to digest organic matter and convert it into rich plant nutrients. Earthworm castings are an extremely valuable source of nitrogen, minerals, and other nutrients. The castings that are left behind after earthworms eat and digest the soil contain five times more nitrogen, seven times more phosphate, and eleven times more potassium than the original soil.

You can obtain earthworms from a compost pile or an old pile of leaves, or you can buy some at any bait and tackle shop. Ask for red wigglers. A couple of handfuls are sufficient to get an entire colony started. The earthworms will go to work producing their weight in castings every twenty-four hours.

Composting Instructions

To get started with your home composting system you will need two or three empty barrels with lids. Drill holes spaced at two-inch intervals all around the sides of the barrels. Place a shallow container of some sort under each barrel. Inverted flat trash can lids work well. It is best if this setup is supported an inch or two off the ground, to allow air circulation underneath. A couple of bricks will do nicely.

When you have harvested some wheatgrass, break up the mats into pieces and place them in a layer in the bottom of the barrel. On top of this layer, spread some vegetable scraps or pulp that has been ejected from your wheatgrass juicer. Following the scraps, put in the earthworms, and cover them with another layer of broken-up mats. (Store scraps and pulp in a sealed container until you have enough mats to cover them.) As you harvest mats, repeat this layering technique, only without adding any more earthworms, until the barrel is full. After each layer is placed in the barrel, cover it with a lid. You can also mix in a handful of lime per barrel if you wish to keep the soil slightly alkaline.

When the compost barrel is full, the decomposition of the mats and vegetable matter intensifies. As long as the barrels are in a warm place, but out of direct sunlight, the compost will develop into rich soil, ready for use in two to three months. If you want to use your compost sooner, in one to two months, remove the lid every week and stir up the contents of the barrel with a shovel. This will expose the inside of the barrel to more oxygen, speeding up the rate of decomposition of the contents.

You will know when the compost is ready by scooping out a shovelful and examining it. If it is crumbly, dark, and without any bad odor or trace of scraps, it is ready. To use the new compost for planting, mix it with 25 percent peat moss.

Compost barrels can be kept in the basement, in a back hallway, on the porch, or in a closet. Even better, purchase some attractive barrels with wheels and tight-fitting lids, and keep them right in your kitchen where they are more accessible. You don't have to worry about any unpleasant odors using this easy composting system. Properly composted earth has a pleasant, woodsy smell.

If more than a few drops of moisture collect under the barrel, the compost is probably too moist. To eliminate any odor that develops, sprinkle a couple of handfuls of lime into the pile, mix it up with a shovel, sprinkle some more lime on the top layer, and cover. To avoid this pitfall, cover scraps totally with mats and avoid adding freshly watered mats to the can. Instead, let them dry out until they are moist, but not wet, and cover the surface with a handful of lime.

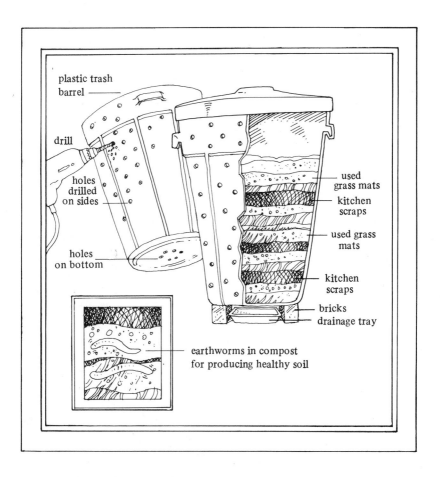

Indoor Composting

Composting Instructions Check List

The main points of my easy composting system are reviewed below:

- Obtain 2 or 3 barrels and drill holes spaced 2 inches apart all around.

- Place broken-up mats in the bottom of a barrel, followed by kitchen scraps and juicer pulp, a few earthworms, and another layer of broken-up mats to cover. When you have additional mats, repeat the layers, without adding more worms, but instead adding a handful of lime (if desired), until the barrel is full. Always re-cover the barrel.

- Let the barrel sit for 2–3 months, at which time your compost will be ready to be mixed with 25 percent peat moss for planting. To speed the composting process, you can stir up the contents of the barrel each week so that the compost will be ready 1 or 2 months later.

If you regularly maintain an outdoor compost pile using a method without animal manures, you may add your mats to it instead. But during the winter months you will be better off if you have a ready supply of compost and a few barrels in progress indoors. At the Hippocrates Institute we send our compost every year or two to our mini-farm in exchange for a fresh supply. The old compost is placed in the gardens, and is reconditioned by the elements. Such a rotation is ideal, as the soil will eventually need to be exposed to the air, rain, and sun, if it is to stay healthy and balanced.

JUICING WHEATGRASS

Since wheatgrass is so fibrous, and its fiber is indigestible by humans, we always use it juiced. You could use your teeth to juice the grass by chewing it and spitting out the pulp, but to get several ounces by this method would wear out your jaw, and your patience! It is far better to purchase a slow-turning juicer made especially for juicing sprouts, greens, soft vegetables, and wheatgrass. Both hand-crank and electric units are available. I recommend the electric model, as to get several ounces of juice using a hand unit is tiring and takes a lot longer. The hand units tend to wind up collecting dust on the closet shelf much more often than the electric models do.

With your electric juicer on, merely place a bunch of cut wheatgrass, about two-thirds of an inch in diameter, tip down into the hole at the top. The juicer will do the rest. A few drops of juice will come out of the front of the juicer, followed by the pulp. The juice itself will come out of the spout on the bottom of the machine. I like to run the pulp through the juicer two or more times to get as much juice out of it as possible. After each use, be sure to take your juicer apart and wash and dry all the parts with a mild, non-detergent soap.

An entire 10″ × 14″ tray of fully mature wheatgrass will produce between seven and ten ounces of wheatgrass juice, depending on the length of the grass and its moisture content. As wheatgrass juice is very volatile, it should be used within twelve hours. With practice, you will learn how much grass to harvest for each use.

If you do not wish to invest in an electric wheatgrass juicer, but still want to use wheatgrass juice, you can try running the grass through a meat grinder (which costs about as much as a hand juicer), and squeeze the mashed pulp through a piece of cheesecloth to extract the juice. However, if you are serious about improving your health, an electric juicer is essential equipment.

Unlike high-speed vegetable juicers, which grind fresh foods and separate the juice from them, a wheatgrass juicer squeezes the juice out slowly. In this way it is able to extract 50 to 98 percent more juice from wheatgrass, greens, sprouts, or soft vegetables than any high-speed machine can. A wheatgrass juicer will be used in extracting fruit and vegetable juices and "green drinks" made from sprouts, greens, and vegetables, which you will need if you wish to perform a wheatgrass fast. The best, and perhaps only, way to purchase a wheatgrass juicer is through the mail (see the Appendix for more information).

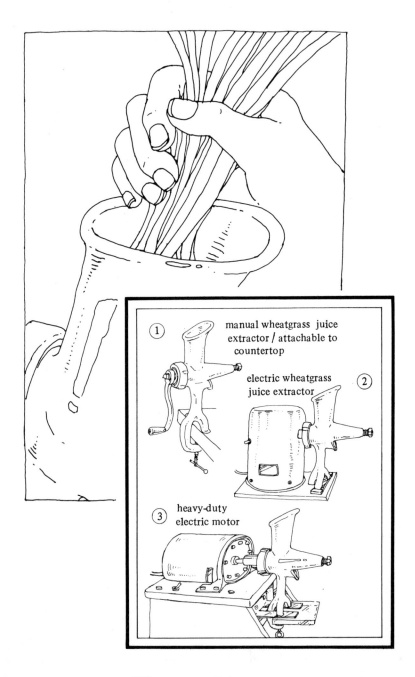

Wheatgrass Juicers

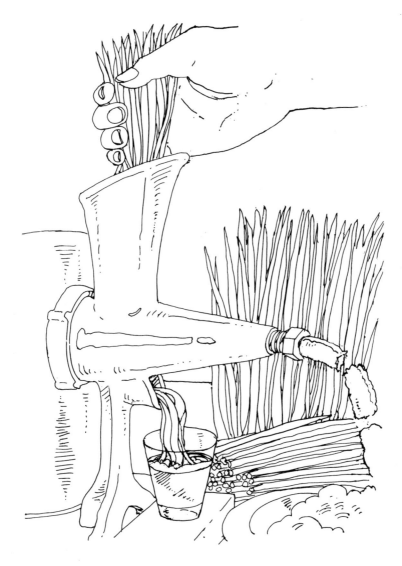

Juicing

If you should have any further questions about setting up an indoor gardening system, or any problems following these instructions, don't hesitate to call the Institute and speak to one of our experts. Better yet, come and stay for the two-week course, and learn by doing while you're here.

8

The Many Uses of Wheatgrass

There is no substitute for good grass any more than there is for water, light and air.

Dr. Charles Schnabel

There are basically two ways to use wheatgrass juice, internally and externally. The internal use of wheatgrass helps to cleanse the blood, organs, and gastrointestinal tract of debris. It stimulates metabolism and bodily enzyme systems in enriching the blood by increasing red blood cell count, and in dilating the blood pathways throughout the body, reducing blood pressure. The thyroid gland is also stimulated and normalized by the use of wheatgrass juice—an important step toward the correction of obesity, indigestion, and a host of other complaints.

As a protective food/medicine, wheatgrass juice is a storehouse of vitamins, minerals, enzymes, amino acids, and oxygen—a great nutritional supplement. Its abundance of alkaline minerals helps it to reduce overacidity in the blood. In addition, it can be used to relieve many internal pains. It has been used successfully to treat peptic ulcers, ulcerative colitis, constipation, diarrhea, and other complaints of the gastrointestinal tract.

FOOD/MEDICINE

The question of how much wheatgrass juice to drink for optimum effect is a little tricky. I have seen enthusiastic students at the Institute drink eight or more ounces of the juice in one sitting their first day there. In some cases, these students felt sick and had to lie down for a while due to the cleansing effects of the juice. This, of course, is not the right way to use wheatgrass juice.

The right way to use wheatgrass juice is in small amounts throughout the course of the day, always on an empty or nearly empty stomach. In general, two to four ounces every day or every other day is sufficient. Slowly sipping small quantities of the juice gives your body an opportunity to get used to its taste and effect. Taking one- to two-ounce drinks straight or mixed with other juices (see the recipes on page 87), and sipping the juice slowly, will help prevent nausea or stomach upset.

On a healing regime, I suggest that you drink one or two ounces up to three or four times a day. If you wish, you may take a day off from drinking wheatgrass juice once in a while. The rest period will enable your body to readjust to the changes it has made, making the juice even more effective the next day.

RECIPES USING WHEATGRASS JUICE

Almost everyone I know uses wheatgrass straight, but a few people have created some marvellous recipes using wheatgrass juice along with other live foods ingredients. I would like to share my favorites with you. In general, you will need three kitchen appliances to make them: a blender with at least three speeds, a high-speed juicer, and a wheatgrass juicer.

Bear in mind that an average tray of fully mature wheatgrass yields between seven and ten ounces of fresh juice. The amount will vary depending on the length and moisture content of the wheatgrass and on whether you run the pulp through the juicer a second or third time. In general, a bunch of wheatgrass one half to two thirds of a inch thick (diameter) will yield about one ounce of juice. Have a two-ounce glass handy to measure the amount of juice for the recipes.

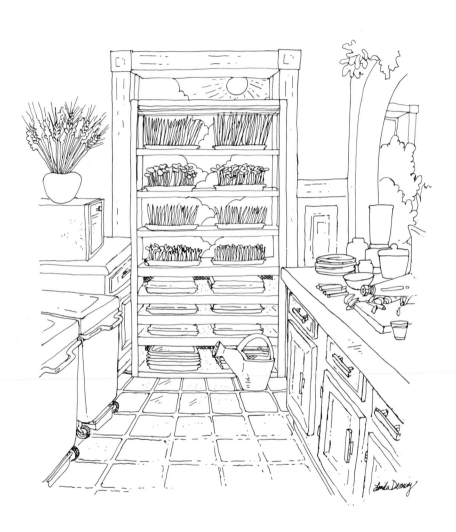

Ann Wigmore's Living Foods Kitchen

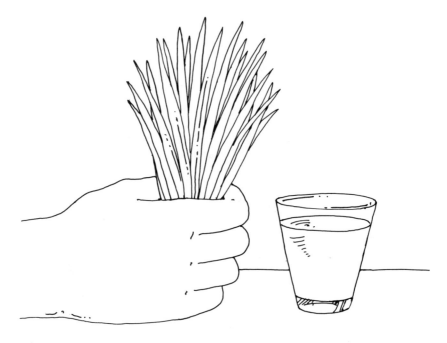

Measuring Juice for Recipes

In recipes where water or ice is listed as an ingredient, use pure spring or filtered water. Vegetables and fruits that have been sprayed or waxed, and those with unedible skins, should be peeled before use. Organically grown fruits and vegetables may not need to be peeled.

The wheatgrass juicer does a good job of making juices from soft vegetables and watery fruits, including leafy greens, sprouts, summer squashes, cucumbers, celery, pineapples, and watermelon, but it does a rather poor job—and is very slow—juicing hard fruits and vegetables. Ingredients such as carrots, beets, apples, and watermelon are best juiced in a high-speed juicer. If, however, a recipe calls for half a beet or apple, or just one carrot, you may want to cut it into bite-sized pieces and use the wheatgrass juicer for convenience. The following recipes each make one serving, approximately eight ounces.

Recipes

Green Drink With Grass

> 1 bunch wheatgrass, about 2/3–3/4
>   inch thick (diameter)
> 3 ounces mixed green and sprout juice
>   (6–7 handfuls of whole ingredients)
> 3 ounces carrot juice (3 medium carrots)

Juice greens, sprouts, and wheatgrass in that order in a wheatgrass juicer. Juice carrots in high-speed machine. Mix juices and serve.

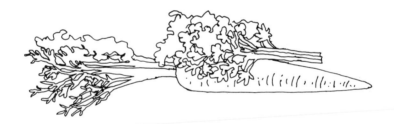

Vegetable Grass Drink

> 3 ounces carrot juice (3 medium carrots)
> 3 ounces celery juice (2 large stalks)
> 1 1/2 ounces wheatgrass juice
> 1/2 ounce parsley juice (five sprigs)

Juice carrots in high-speed machine, and other ingredients in wheatgrass juicer. Mix and serve.

Wheat-Beet Juice
---

1 1/2 ounces wheatgrass juice
1 ounce beet juice (1/2 medium beet)
6 ounces cucumber juice (1/2 large
cucumber)

Juice ingredients in wheatgrass juicer, stir, and serve.

Wheatgrass Cocktail
---

1 1/2 ounces wheatgrass juice
6 ounces fresh apple juice
(2 medium apples)

Mix wheatgrass juice and apple juice in a glass and serve.

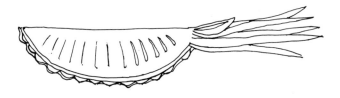

Wheatgrasshopper

---

1 1/2 ounces wheatgrass juice
6 ounces pineapple juice (1/4 pineapple)
2 ice cubes
3 leaves fresh mint

Blend ingredients together at high speed for thirty seconds, and serve.

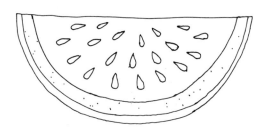

Wheatgrass-Rind Juice

---

1 1/2 ounces wheatgrass juice
6 ounces watermelon rind juice
  (1 piece, 3″ × 8″)

Cut red meat from watermelon, and set aside for later use.
Juice rind in high-speed juicer. Mix juices and serve.

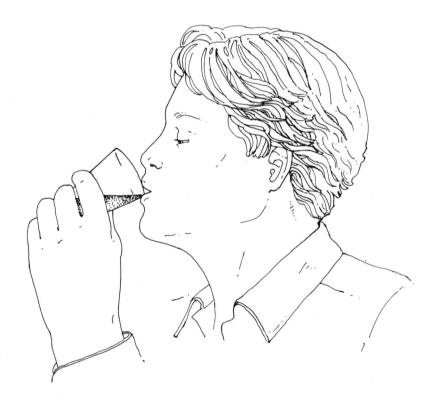

Wheatgrass Juice—A Refreshing Drink

WHEATGRASS JUICE BRINGS RELIEF

While wheatgrass juice makes a refreshing and enlivening drink, you may not always want to use it in that way. You may want to chew or gargle it, for example, to freshen stale breath or to relieve a sore throat. If chewed and applied to a sore tooth or to the gums, it will help reduce swelling and pain. Rubbed into the gums on a regular basis, it can help remedy pyorrhea and bleeding.

An effective eye wash for the relief of eyestrain and itchiness can be made from finely strained wheatgrass juice. Apply the juice with a dropper or purchase an eyecup at a drugstore. When placed in the ear with a dropper, strained wheatgrass juice helps reduce the pressure and discomfort of many an earache. If drops are inserted into the nasal passages and inhaled, it will help cleanse and open sinuses.

When using wheatgrass juice in these sensitive areas, you may experience a temporary worsening of symptoms. Your eyes may be even more itchy and red or your sinuses may clog further, but be assured that these reactions are temporary and will diminish greatly a few minutes later. At the Institute, we regard such reactions as a positive sign—that is, as an indication that the body is being cleansed of unwholesome substances. However, you may try using less wheatgrass juice next time, and diluting it with some water. Also try using wheatgrass in the many other ways it can be used outside the body. If reactions persist, discontinue use.

In addition, I have found through personal experience that wheatgrass juice can be used as a douche to help eliminate cystitis, vaginal infections, odors, and itching.

WHEATGRASS IMPLANTS

Another way in which wheatgrass is used internally at the Hippocrates Institute is as a rectal implant or retention enema. In many people, the lower bowel has become a dumping ground, its walls encrusted with debris and bulging with bubble-like diverticula. The use of an enema to cleanse the colon, followed by a wheatgrass implant, helps stimulate peristaltic activity of the muscles that contract the colon wall. This helps to loosen deposits that may be seen later (after defecation) in the form of hardened black material and ropes or lumps of mucus. In addition, the high magnesium content of wheatgrass juice draws fat out of the colon wall and the liver.

In an implant, fresh wheatgrass is inserted into the rectum and retained there for about twenty minutes before being expelled. Implants are especially helpful in the case of illness, serious or otherwise, as they stimulate a rapid cleansing of the lower bowel. In my opinion, wheatgrass implants are safer than the coffee enemas used by many health clinics, because wheatgrass does not introduce unwanted caffeine. (As a matter of fact, wheatgrass implants introduce many important nutrients to the body.)

All this talk about wheatgrass implants may leave you feeling a bit squeamish. If you have a psychological barrier against doing implants and enemas, try to remind yourself of their purpose—to reverse damage and draw out accumulations of debris that may be lurking inside you. If you can bring yourself to use these cleansing techniques, you will find relief and a sense of internal cleanliness that is refreshing. Besides, the removal of toxic and morbid matter from the colon is essential to healing.

If you are planning to use wheatgrass implants, it is best to perform an enema before you do so. Early in the morning is probably the best time to do both; however, if this is not possible or if repetition is desired, early afternoon and evening are also good times.

How to Take a Wheatgrass Implant

To use wheatgrass juice implants as a purge, simply fill a sterilized infant enema syringe with one to two ounces of fresh juice and insert it into the rectum. A couple of minutes later, the bowels will move hurriedly. Try another one to two ounce implant and also let it out if it wants to come. The second attempt will probably carry more fecal matter with it. A third implant, of two to six ounces, will usually be retained with ease. Hold it until you feel the urge to eliminate, generally about twenty minutes later. There is no danger of reabsorbing toxins if you have purged the colon first with other implants or enemas. You may even be surprised to find that your body has absorbed all the juice after twenty minutes.

Wheatgrass implants are especially effective in conjunction with the wheatgrass fast, which I will discuss in the next chapter.

OTHER USES FOR WHEATGRASS JUICE

There are many ways you can use wheatgrass juice externally. Applied to the skin, it can help eliminate itching almost immediately. It will soothe sunburned skin, and also act as a disinfectant. As a beauty treatment, it will help tighten loose and sagging skin. Rubbed into the scalp before a shampoo, it will help mend damaged hair and alleviate itchy, scaly scalp conditions and irritations. Try leaving the juice on your scalp for a couple of hours before washing it off.

Every household should have some wheatgrass juice for soothing and healing cuts, burns, scrapes, rashes, poison ivy, athlete's foot, insect bites, boils, sores, open ulcers, tumors, and so on. Of course, the juice won't stay fresh in a first aid kit, but you can always soak a lump of wheatgrass pulp in fresh juice and apply it directly to the affected area, or pour fresh juice onto a bandage, apply it where needed, and cover the area with a clean, dry cloth. The poultice should be replaced every two to four hours. Clean the area with castile soap and let it "breathe" a few minutes before reapplying the poultice. One way to enjoy *all* of the beneficial effects of wheatgrass juice is to add some to your bath water, and settle in for a nice, long soak.

As a sleep aid, merely place a tray of living wheatgrass near the head of your bed. It will enhance the oxygen in the air and generate healthful negative ions to help you sleep more soundly. I have seen remarkable results when insomniacs have placed just one or two trays of wheatgrass by the bedside.

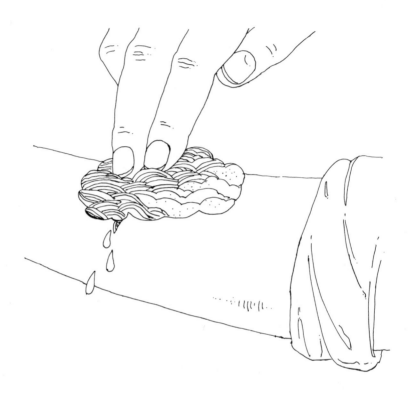

Wheatgrass as a Poultice

Over the years, many pets, including cats, dogs, birds, monkeys, and gerbils, have benefited from the use of wheatgrass and its juice. Even healthy pets nibble grass to get roughage (fiber), which is lacking in most prepared pet foods. If your pet seems to be ill, try chopping some fresh grass into its food. (Chop it finely if you are feeding a dog or a cat, because these animals do not chew their food well.) You may also be able to give your pet wheatgrass juice either in its drinking water or with a dropper. If all else fails, try rubbing a small amount of wheatgrass juice onto your pet's fur. In most cases the animal will lick it off. If your pet does not perk up within a few days, consult a veterinarian.

Earlier I discussed how wheatgrass juice changes tap water by neutralizing certain harmful elements in it. Keep in mind, however, that adding wheatgrass juice is no replacement for proper filtering and home refiltering of municipal water. Instead use the improved-quality tap water to grow sprouts, wheatgrass, greens, and houseplants, or, as mentioned above, to feed your pets.

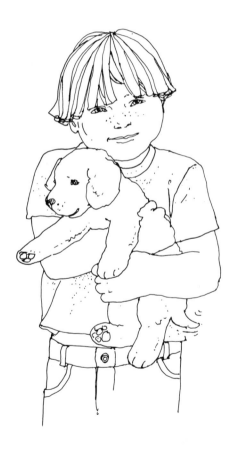

A Happy Pet

9

The Wheatgrass Fast:
For Cleansing, Healing,
and Super Nutrition

When freshly made into a drink, chlorophyll contains
synthesized sunshine, plus the electric current necessary for
the revitalization of the body—and it will open up areas of the
brain that man as yet knows nothing about.

Rev. J.L. Moran

Over the years many books and articles have been writtten on
the benefits of fasting as a means of eliminating toxins from
the body and allowing the digestive system to rest and repair
itself. What the writers don't mention, however, is that
extended fasts, despite the rewards they offer, can be
dangerous. My own opinion is that long periods of abstaining
from all nutrition are unnecessary and too harsh for the average person.

An ideal compromise is the wheatgrass fast. It offers the
satisfaction of fasting and cleansing the body in one of the
quickest ways possible, and does so with complete safety. During the three-day fast, you will drink not only wheatgrass juice,
but highly nourishing and palatable green drinks extracted
from sprouts, baby greens, and some vegetables, as well.
Sweetened lemon water and Rejuvelac, a fermented wheat-
berry drink I developed over twenty years ago, can also be
used.

Whereas water fasting may leave you feeling weak, tired, and disoriented at times, on the wheatgrass fast most people feel good enough to perform their normal activities.

One of the main advantages of the wheatgrass fast is that it combines perhaps the most nutritious liquids known, wheatgrass juice and green drinks. In fact, I estimate that three 8-ounce green drinks and two 4-ounce servings of wheatgrass juice contain about sixty grams of vitamins, minerals, and protein, more than adequate for an active adult, based on the Recommended Daily Allowances established by the U.S. Food and Drug Administration.

The only thing the wheatgrass fast may be short on is calories. As long as you end the fast after three days, the reduced calorie intake will probably do you good because your body will be forced to burn waste and excess weight as fuel for energy. In fact, the average weight loss on the three-day wheatgrass fast is between four and ten pounds.

PREPARING FOR THE WHEATGRASS FAST

The wheatgrass fast is not for everyone. If you are at all apprehensive about doing it, for any reason whatsoever, you're probably not ready for it—and you may never be. You can, however, cleanse and repair your body in the same way, only more slowly, merely by following the Hippocrates Diet and using wheatgrass juice. For most people, especially those with health problems, and older folks, it is probably best to add wheatgrass and raw foods to the regular diet before attempting a fast.

Also, if you are squeamish about enemas or implants, the fast may not be for you. More than any other precaution, I feel that daily enemas are essential during the fast. So much sticky mucus and toxic matter can be dumped into the colon, that its efficient removal can make the difference between feeling terrible and having more energy than you ever had before.

Finally, for maximum benefit from the three-day fast, you must have the opportunity to rest. Set aside a time without any appointments or other scheduling demands. You may find a holiday weekend ideal for this.

PHYSICAL CHANGES DURING THE FAST

When I first began my work in the health field more than thirty years ago, I was terrified of what many alternative health educators called the "healing crisis"—a dismal period of nausea, vomiting, diarrhea, boils, low energy, and enforced bed rest, which—if you survived—would end your health problems forever. Since then my fear has been replaced by confidence and common sense. If you take meat, potatoes, white bread, vegetables, eggs, cheese, fruit, ice cream, junk foods, coffee, alcohol, sodas, and milk away from a person, and give him only water to drink for a month, a healing crisis is inevitable. I have had to nurse many well-intentioned individuals back to health after they tried this cold plunge route. Once their healing crises abated, usually after a few days, the super energy and dynamism they had been promised as a result of their suffering never came about. Some of them would have been happy just to get back the amount of energy they had before the fast, such was the draining effect the crisis had on their bodies.

Fortunately, a healing crisis isn't inevitable or even desirable. Even if you could suffer your way to better health, it would hardly be worth the effort since you can achieve the same results while being good to your body. Why did the idea of the beneficial healing crisis arise? Deep down inside we tell ourselves that we must suffer to redeem ourselves from the wrong foods and lack of exercise in our past. Rubbish.

Many people have benefited from the wheatgrass fast, but, in all my years in the health field, I have never seen the so-called healing crisis occur as long as my instructions were followed in a common-sense way. For example, I recommend one to four ounces of wheatgrass juice, three times per day for three days. More than once, individuals attending the Institute have exceeded this amount. One person I remember drank nearly a quart of wheatgrass over a two-hour period; for the next two days he couldn't touch his food, slept nearly half the day, and stayed close to the bathroom at all times. Since wheatgrass is a medicine as well as a food, common sense dictates that you shouldn't take a quart in two hours, or even ten ounces four times a day for a week! Wheatgrass is non-toxic in any amount, but more isn't necessarily better.

The important point is that you needn't journey to hell and back again to be well. The "inevitable" healing crisis will probably never get a foothold in your body if you use common sense and follow my recommendations.

PERFORMING THE FAST

Try not to push yourself too hard during the three days of the fast. Keep the days totally empty of appointments or errands and instead read, do light exercise, work in the yard, go for a stroll, bask on the beach, or whatever—but relax. You may feel the urge to sleep a lot. As long as you drink the recommended three quarts of liquid each day, extra sleep will do your body good.

Every morning of the fast, and again in the evening if you wish, perform a simple water enema to cleanse the colon. Follow the morning enema with a wheatgrass implant. You can take four or more implants throughout the day, using up to six ounces of wheatgrass juice for each one.

Drink one to four ounces of wheatgrass juice straight, three times per day. Alternatively, you can dilute the juice with water or even add it to a green drink. However, drinking it straight is probably the best ideas in terms of digestibility. Space the wheatgrass drinks out well during the day. You may want to take one in the morning, another at noon, and the last one at dinnertime. Follow all the wheatgrass drinks with an eight- to twelve-ounce green drink (see page 108) about half an hour later.

When you are thirsty between the three meals of wheatgrass and green drinks, drink lemon water, lightly sweetened with raw honey, or Rejuvelac (with a little honey in it if you like). Drink a total of three quarts of liquid each day.

BREAKING THE FAST

Following the fast, it is important for you to let your body adjust to solid foods slowly. There is a tendency for fasters to wake up on the morning of the fourth day and eat everything in sight! Unfortunately, if you give in to that urge, you will probably undo all the good you have just done—and you may become sick to your stomach. It is much better to break the fast with a breakfast (or dinner, if you are breaking it at night) of fresh fruits.

Choose one or two fruits and eat a moderate amount. For example, a couple of apples and a handful of grapes, or a pear and some cherries. For the rest of the day, or the next two or three meals, you may eat salads with all kinds of sprouts, greens, and raw vegetables. Use dressings made from vegetables, seeds, or avocados, rather than from oil, vinegar, garlic, and the like. You can have the first salad about three or four hours after the fruit meal, and after a day or so of fruits and raw salads you may begin to eat other foods as well.

I recommend, however, that you continue to make fresh fruits and raw salads, along with green juices, a part of your diet. Gradually add more of them to your daily fare, or, even better, adopt the Hippocrates living foods diet. Whatever you do, don't begin to eat heavy cooked meals with animal foods immediately following the fast, as they will drain your energy level tremendously and may cause constipation and cravings for more and different foods—especially the ones that I urge you never to eat again.

FASTING DO'S AND DON'TS

You may have to adjust the wheatgrass fast to your own needs and desires. This section will give you some guidelines on how to do so. The recommendation to drink three quarts of liquid per day, for example, is vital to the fasting process and should not be ignored. The way of breaking the fast is also important, along with daily enemas, and preferably implants as well. On the other hand, one thing you may choose to vary is the number of days you fast. If you want, you can fast for one day, two days, or the full three days.

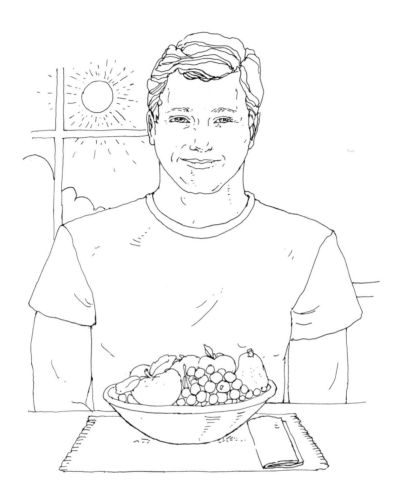

Breakfast Meal After Fasting

If halfway through the first day you feel terrible and think that it will be too stressful for you to continue at this time, simply break the fast with a piece of fresh fruit. Nobody is going to point a finger at you and tell you that you failed. Just the fact that you began the fast in the first place makes you anything but a failure.

In the same way, if you just can't manage to get down all the wheatgrass or green drinks each day of the fast, don't despair. You can substitute other kinds of fresh juices. A modified wheatgrass fast, using most or some but not all of the recommended green juices, will also be beneficial. If the fasting process is going to be one long punishment for you, it's better to change it to suit your needs, or to abandon it altogether.

To some degree, during any type of fast, the blood pools in the abdominal region of the body. There is nothing bad about having more blood in this area, but it does mean that there is less blood in the head. This could cause a little dizziness if you attempt too many quick starts. So exercise care in your activities while you are fasting.

Many people experience surges of energy during one or all of the days. They have an urge to set new records for the number of miles they can walk or hours they can work. Try not to overdo it. Instead be moderate and channel your energy into the internal housecleaning that is occurring. Some mild exercise will be beneficial, but hours of walking or working will not.

Also, if possible, stay close to home. Traveling during fasting isn't advised, especially driving long distances. In certain ways the mind and reflexes may not be as sharp during the fast. Caution should be your guide. If you can, spend lots of time outdoors in the sun, tinkering in your garden, and so on. Sunlight will stimulate various body cleansing processes. For this reason, I suggest that you begin the fast in warmer weather.

Don't drink more of the wheatgrass or green drinks than you feel you can handle at any one time. Their cleansing activity can cause you to lose your appetite for them after a day or so. If this happens, it is better not to force them down. Try coming back to them a couple of hours later and in the meantime sip Rejuvelac, lemon water, or carrot juice.

Because of the need for rest and freedom from schedules during the wheatgrass fast, I don't allow it to be performed by guests at the Institute any more. After years of observation I have learned that the Hippocrates Diet is ideal for the kind of activities and the busy schedule at the Institute. If your job or lifestyle makes it difficult to set aside three undemanding days, concentrate on improving your diet from day to day, instead of attempting the wheatgrass fast.

A TYPICAL DAY ON THE
WHEATGRASS FAST

The following summary of a typical day on the wheatgrass fast
may serve as a handy reference guide.

- Begin each day of the fast with an enema, followed by an
  implant or two, using up to 6 ounces of fresh wheatgrass
  juice in each one.

- Take one 8-ounce glass of lemon water or Rejuvelac, with a
  little honey if desired. Follow this with wheatgrass juice a
  half hour later, and a green drink another half hour after
  that (see recipes for green drinks on page 108).

- In between breakfast and lunchtime, you may take another
  wheatgrass implant and drink another glass of Rejuvelac or
  lemon water if desired. Follow with a lunch of wheatgrass
  juice and another green drink. Have the same for dinner.

- Up to four wheatgrass implants can be used throughout the
  day. One before bed is especially helpful for sound sleep.

- Get plenty of rest and relaxation. Do some light stretching
  and walking, spend some time out of doors, and don't force
  yourself to follow a schedule or meet any deadlines.

- Break the fast after one, two, or three days with a meal of
  fresh fruit followed several hours later with a salad made of
  sprouts, greens, and fresh vegetables, with an oil-free dress-
  ing.

MAKING GREEN DRINKS AND
REJUVELAC

Making Rejuvelac and green drinks for use during the fast or
at any other time is simple. Using a wheatgrass juicer, juice
several cups of sprouts, sunflower and buckwheat greens, and
other vegetables, such as peppers, cucumbers, celery, and carrots. Recipes for a few of my favorite green drinks, particularly suited for use on the wheatgrass fast, are included at the

end of this chapter. Each of them will make approximately eight ounces of juice.

Rejuvelac

To make Rejuvelac, you will need a clean quart-sized jar and a piece of screening or netting (made of a non-toxic material such as nylon) to cover it with, a couple of handfuls of whole wheatberries, some spring or filtered water, and patience. The starter batch will need to ferment for about forty-eight hours.

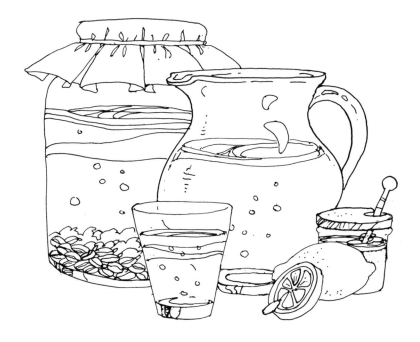

Rejuvelac

Soft pastry wheatberries are best, but other varieties will do as long as they are organically grown. The soft pastry wheatberries are frequently lighter in color than the hard winter varieties which are recommended for home growing, but otherwise closely resemble them. If you wish, you may use day-old sprouted wheat to make Rejuvelac.

Start by washing a cup of whole wheatberries in a jar of cool water. Discard any berries that float to the surface. Place the washed berries in a quart-sized jar. If you use sprouted berries, simply rinse them before placing them in the jar. Fill the jar with water, cover, and allow the mixture to sit undisturbed for forty-eight hours. Then strain out the liquid Rejuvelac, leaving the berries and sediment in the jar.

Refill the same jar with water and set aside once more, this time for only twenty-four hours. Pour off the Rejuvelac, again saving the berries, and refill the jar for the third and last time with water. Allow it to ferment for another twenty-four hours, pour off the Rejuvelac, and this time discard the original wheatberries. That's all there is to it. Start one or two batches on different days so that you will always have some Rejuvelac ready to use. It should taste tart, not too sour, and may be enjoyed with a little lemon juice or honey for variety. Unused Rejuvelac will keep in the refrigerator for two to three days.

Recipes

When making green drinks, cut the vegetables in the largest-size pieces that will fit in your juicer. The only exception to this is if a recipe calls for a small quantity of a hard vegetable, such as one carrot or half a beet, and you are going to juice it in a wheatgrass juicer. In this case it is best to cut the vegetables into bite-sized pieces before juicing them. Where larger volumes of juice are needed, for instance, if you are making drinks for ten people, juicing hard vegetables in a high-speed juicer will save time.

Like wheatgrass juice, green drinks should be used as soon as possible after they are prepared. However, they can be kept refrigerated for about twelve hours if it is not possible for you to use them immediately. After twelve hours they should be discarded.

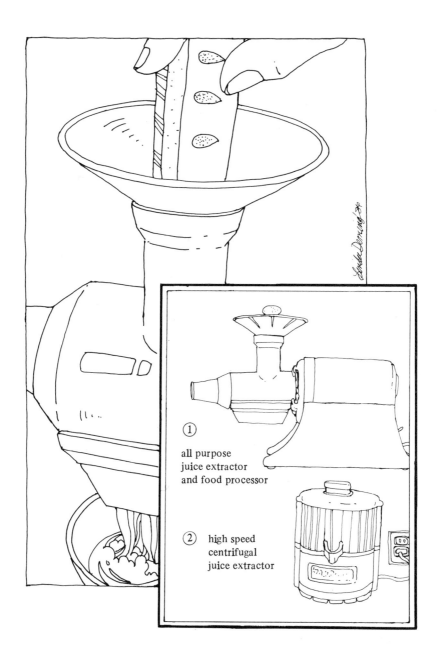

1. all purpose
   juice extractor
   and food processor

2. high speed
   centrifugal
   juice extractor

Vegetable/Fruit Juicers

Basic Green Drink

---

4 cups alfalfa and/or other sprouts
4 cups sunflower and buckwheat greens
1/2 cup carrots
1/2 cup sweet red pepper
1/4 cup parsley
1 cup cucumber

Juice ingredients in wheatgrass juicer and serve immediately.

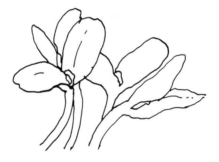

Sunflower Greens

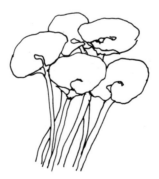

Buckwheat Greens

Garden Green Drink

---

4 cups sprouts
4 cups greens
2 cups kale or collard greens
1 cup celery
1/2 cup sauerkraut

Juice ingredients (sauerkraut last) in wheatgrass juicer and serve.

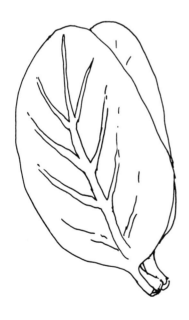

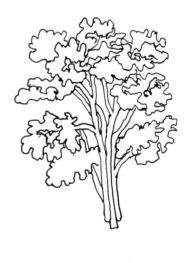

Collard Greens   **Kale**

Green Power Cocktail
---

4 cups sprouts
4 cups greens
1 cup celery
1 cup kale
1 cup beets
1/2 cup wheatgrass

Juice ingredients (wheatgrass last) in wheatgrass juicer and serve.

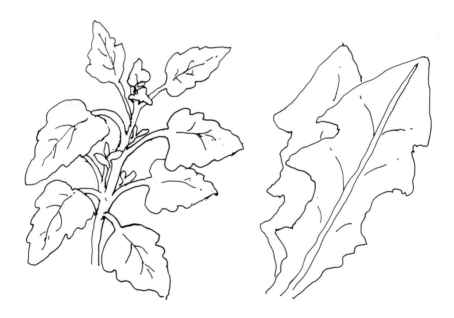

Lamb's-Quarters   **Dandelion Greens**

Spring Green Drink

---

4 cups sprouts
4 cups greens
1 cup lamb's-quarters
1/2 cup dandelion greens
1/4 cup scallion
1 cup carrots

Juice ingredients in wheatgrass juicer and serve.

See also Recipes Using Wheatgrass Juice, pages 87–90.

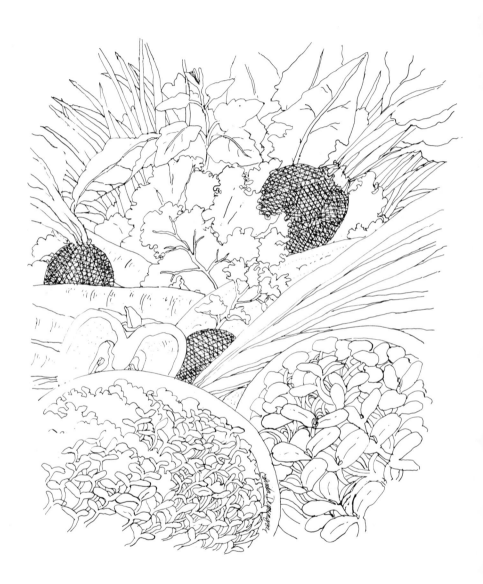

An Abundance of Vegetables

Epilogue

Welcome To The
New Green Revolution

*Bad men live that they may eat and drink, whereas good
men eat and drink to live.*

Socrates

I often recall the early days when I began experimenting with
wheatgrass. I was always amused by the struggles I had trying
to uproot clods of grass from the garden. Little did I realize
that the power that fought my tugging fingers could transform
and regenerate the human body.

Now I know better. After years of research and travel, I am
convinced that what we need most today is a fundamental
change in eating and lifestyle to give us the stronger, healthier
bodies that will overcome the many other problems facing the
world today.

For years the western world has been gambling with human
health in a great experiment that has us eating more than 50
percent of our food from packages and cans. About three
thousand different chemical additives are used in processing
our foods, despite convincing evidence that they can affect the
delicate electrochemical balance in the brain and nervous system. Fortunately, you and I have a say in the matter. We can
gain more control over our diets, our health, and our lives by

making simple changes in the way we live. Growing a percentage of our own food at home in the form of baby greens and sprouts can give us control over at least a portion of what we eat. We can then select the rest from the fresh foods sold at farm stands, natural foods stores, and supermarkets. Wheatgrass juice will help to compensate for the nutritional deficiencies in modern foods, and protect us from pollution and other physical and environmental stresses.

Wheatgrass is not going to cure the ills of the world, but it is an important element in what I call the new green revolution—a greater emphasis, on the part of people everywhere, on working with nature to prevent illness before it takes hold. Until quite recently, our society was moving in the wrong direction, especially in the areas of food production and processing. But it is not too late for us to recognize our mistake and to embrace nature's idea of nourishment in wheatgrass and live foods.

Young blades of wheatgrass are a storehouse of essential vitamins, minerals, and enzymes. The amount of vitamins A and C in wheatgrass juice compares favorably with the vitamin content of many common fruits and garden vegetables. In addition, wheatgrass juice contains optimum amounts of the B-complex vitamins, Vitamin E, and minerals such as calcium, iron, sodium, and potassium. Fresh wheatgrass juice supplies these nutrients in a form in which they may be readily utilized by the body. Moreover, when wheatgrass juice is used fresh, it is full of living enzyme energy that can promote healthy blood circulation and rejuvenate aging cells.

In animal nutrition, wheatgrass juice has already proven itself to be miracle worker. No other plant has the ability to ensure generation after generation of healthy litters in herbivorous animals all by itself. And no other potent food suitable for human consumption is as inexpensive to produce. Spirulina and chlorella, bee pollen, and other supplemental health foods may be chemically potent, but compared to fresh wheatgrass juice, they are low in vitality, and much more costly. Vitamin and mineral supplements are also costly, and often unsafe.

Many of us have poor eating habits and many of us have come to believe certain health myths fostered by our society. Health is not bestowed upon us by our parents or grandparents. While good genes are helpful, most of us have no one to blame for poor health but ourselves. It is a tragic mistake for you to give up responsibility for your day-to-day health or to lay the blame for it on somebody else's doorstep.

If you have ever felt completely in control of your health, clear and clean inside, full of energy, awake, confident, and relaxed, you know what a wonderful feeling it is. I can't promise you that wheatgrass juice alone will make you feel like this, but it will help, especially if you make a commitment to learn more about the other elements of a healthful lifestyle. In *The Hippocrates Diet and Health Program* and in my other books, I have discussed these concepts in detail.

In this book, I have tried to present an overview of the philosophy behind the use of wheatgrass and to describe its practical applications. If you have further questions about growing or using wheatgrass feel free to write or call the Hippocrates Institute in Boston.

I hope that you will join me and thousands of others in the new green revolution. Adding wheatgrass and live foods to your diet can bring you renewed confidence and vitality. A small investment in time and effort will give you a treasure more precious than all the gold and silver in the world—the knowledge that you have done all you can towards perfect health, long life, and peace of mind.

Appendix

If you have any questions about growing or
using wheatgrass, feel free to write or call
the Hippocrates Institute. Information about
live foods equipment, supplies, health aids,
the Hippocrates Program, and the other
books in the Hippocrates Health Series, is
also available.

Hippocrates Health Institute
25 Exeter Street
Boston, MA 02116
(617) 267-9525

Selected References

"Anti-Cancer Effects of Young Barley Grass Leaves," translation of article from newspaper in Hokkaido, Japan. August 29, 1979.

"The Anti-Mutagenic Action of Young Barley Grass Leaves," translation of article from newspaper in Yomiuri, Japan. April 13, 1980.

Calloway, D.H., Calhoun, W.K., and Munson, A.K. "Further Studies on Reduction of X-Radiation Mortality of Guinea Pigs by Plant Materials." *Armed Forces Report*, 12 (1961): 61.

Diet, Nutrition, and Cancer. Washington, DC: National Academy Press, 1982.

Duplan, J.F. "Influence of Dietary Regimen on Radiosensitivity of the Guinea Pig," *Compt Rend Acad Sci*, 236 (1953): 424.

Gillie, Oliver, "New Clues to Cancer." *Times* (London). January, 1977.

Gordon, P. "Free Radicals and the Aging Process," in *Theoretical Aspects of Aging*, M. Rockstein, ed. New York: Academic Press, 1974.

Grant, James, "Of Mice and Men," *Barron's National Financial Weekly*, June 11, 1979.

Gurskin, Benjamine, in the *American Journal of Surgery*, 49 (1940): 49.

Hagiwara, Yoshihide. *Green Barley Essence: A Surprising Source of Health*. Tokyo, Japan: Association of Green and Health Distributors, 1981.

Hoover, Richard. *Cereal Grasses: A Complete Food*. Natick, MA: V.E. Irons Company, 1972.

Hotta, Yasuo. *Preliminary Report on How the Juice of Young Green Barley Grass Plants Can Normalize and Rejuvenate Cells and Tissue, Can Repair Damaged DNA, Restore Cellular Activity, and Prevent Aging of Tissue*. Carson, CA: Green Foods Corporation, 1981.

Hughes, J.H., and Latner, A.L. "Chlorophyll and Hemoglobin Regeneration After Hemorrhage," *Journal of Physiology*, 86 (1936): 388.

Hunsberger, Eydie Mae, and Loeffler, Chris. *How I Conquered Cancer Naturally*. San Diego: Production House, 1975.

Jensen, Bernard. *Chlorophyll Magic From Living Plant Life*. Escondidi, CA: Jensen Publications, 1973.

Kohler, G.O., Elvehjem, C.A., and Hart, E.B., "Growth Stimulating Properties of Grass Juice," *Science*, 83 (1936): 445.

Kohler, G.O., Elvehjem, C.A., and Hart, E.B., "The Relation of the 'Grass Juice Factor' to Guinea Pig Nutrition," *Journal of Nutrition*, 15 (1938): 445.

Kubota, Kazuhiko. "Anti-Inflammatory Effects of Green Barley Juice," address to annual meeting of the Japanese Pharmaceutical Society, April, 1980.

Lai, Chiu-Nan. "Chlorophyll: The Active Factor in Wheat Sprout Extract Inhibiting the Metabolic Activation of Carcinogens in vitro," *Nutrition and Cancer*, 1 (1978): 3.

Miller, Lois M. "Chlorophyll for Healing," *Science Newsletter*, March 15, 1941.

Morgan, W.S. "The Clinical Use of Chlorophyll," *Guthrie Clinical Bulletin*, 16 (1947): 94.

Morishita, Keiichi, and Hotta, Kaneo. *Medicine of Chlorophyll*. Tokyo, Japan: Association of Life Sciences Publishers, 1974 (translation).

Patek, A.J. "Chlorophyll and Regeneration of the Blood," *Archives of Internal Medicine*, 57 (1936): 76.

Patek, A.J., and Minot, E.M. "Bile Pigment and Hemoglobin Regeneration," *American Journal of Medical Science*, 188 (1934): 206.

Pearson, Durk, and Shaw, Sandy. *Life Extension*. Denver, CO: Nutri Books, 1983.

Pike, Arnold. "Special Report on Green Barley Grass," *Let's Live*, March, 1982.

Rafsky, H.A., and Krieger, C.I. "Treatments of Intestinal Diseases with Solutions of Watersoluble Chlorophyll," *Review of Gastroenterology*, 15 (1948): 549.

Robinson, Arthur. "Living Foods and Cancer," *Hippocrates Newsletter*, March, 1984.

Rudolph, Theodore, *Nature's Green Magic*. Los Angeles: Rudolph Publishers, 1972.

Saunders, C.W., in *Proceedings of the Society for Experimental Biology*, 23 (1925): 788.

Schass, Alex. *Diet, Crime, and Delinquency*. New York: Simon and Schuster, 1980.

Schnabel, Charles. "Grass: The Forgiveness of Nature," *Acres USA*, January, 1980.

Smith, J. "Remarks Upon the History, Chemistry, Toxicity, and Antibacterial Properties of Watersoluble Chlorophyll Derivatives as

Therapeutic Agents," *American Journal of Medical Science,* 207 (1944): 649.

Spector, Harry, and Calloway, Doris H. "Reduction of X-Radiation Mortality by Cabbage and Broccoli," *Proceedings of the Society for Experimental Biological Medicine,* 100 (1959): 405.

U.S. Department of Health, Education, and Welfare. *Current Estimates from the Health Interview Survey,* National Center for Health Statistics, Series 10, pubn. no. 72 (1972).

Warburg, Otto. "On the Origin of Cancer Cells," *Science,* 123 (1956).

Young, R.W., and Beregi, J.S., "Use of Chlorophyll in the Care of Geriatric Patients," *Journal of the American Geriatric Society.* 28/1 (1980): 46-47.

Index